Mediatization of
Physical Activity

Mediatization of Physical Activity

Media Saturation and Technologies

Katarzyna Kopecka-Piech

LEXINGTON BOOKS
Lanham • Boulder • New York • London

Published by Lexington Books
An imprint of The Rowman & Littlefield Publishing Group, Inc.
4501 Forbes Boulevard, Suite 200, Lanham, Maryland 20706
www.rowman.com

6 Tinworth Street, London SE11 5AL, United Kingdom

British Library Cataloguing in Publication Information Available

Library of Congress Cataloging-in-Publication Data Available

ISBN 978-1-4985-8470-8 (cloth : alk. paper)
ISBN 978-1-4985-8471-5 (electronic)

∞™ The paper used in this publication meets the minimum requirements of
American National Standard for Information Sciences—Permanence of Paper
for Printed Library Materials, ANSI/NISO Z39.48-1992.

Printed in the United States of America

Contents

Acknowledgments

This book would not have come to life if it were not for the help of many generous and talented people. First and foremost, I would like to thank my colleagues from the Department of Sports Communication and Management at the University School of Physical Education in Wrocław, and in particular Gabriel Łasiński for inspiring me to get engaged in this topic.

This project would not be possible without the financial and organizational support from the Wrocław Academic Center by the Municipality of Wrocław, under whose auspices I completed a project called "SMS—Sports' Media Saturation" which served as a springboard for my further research in mediatization of physical activity. I also want to thank Bartłomiej Skowron (Warsaw University of Technology) for the words of encouragement and unwavering support during the course of work on this project as well as my colleagues from the Academy of Young Scholars and Artists: Justyna Ziółkowska (SWPS University of Social Sciences and Humanities in Warsaw), Adam Mrozowicki (University of Wroclaw), and Grzegorz Kozdraś (University of Wroclaw) for offering consultancy and participant training on qualitative and quantitative methodologies, respectively. I want to thank my students Agata Ludzis-Todorov, Ilona Cięszczyk, Michał Krzesiński, Julia Cypryańska, Natalia Bujko, Julia Zdobylak, and Konrad Słomiński for their engagement in the entire research process from its inception to obtaining survey data and carrying out the interviews.

I am also deeply indebted to the management of the Faculty of Sports Science at the University School of Physical Education in Wrocław, who financially contributed to the empirical aspect of the project and provided the assistance of Aleksandra Leszczyńska, who obtained a significant part of data from interviews and observations.

I am grateful for the support of Iwona Żuk from Ipsylon, a data analysis company, who processed and prepared statistical data in textual and graphic forms and always provided professional support and worthy insights. Also, I would like to thank Jarosław Drapała (Wroclaw University of Technology) and Adam Płoszaj (University of Warsaw) for invaluable data consultancy.

I also want to thank the organizers and participants of seminars and conferences where I had the opportunity to present subsequent results of my research and obtain critical feedback and pertinent advice. I owe special thanks to Göran Bolin (Södertörn University) for constructive remarks on the book while it was in progress.

I owe special thanks to the management of the Faculty of Letters at the University of Wrocław for financing the text work on this book. I thank Arkadiusz Lewicki, the director of The Institute of Journalism and Social Communication, for his unyielding confidence and kind support in the last stages of my project.

I also appreciate all anonymous participants who generously offered their time to engage in this project—without you, this book would not have had a chance to exist.

Moreover, I am obliged to Agata Hamilton, the book's translator, and Ramona Ślusarczyk, a lecturer at Newcastle University, for their editing and proofreading of my work.

Last but not least, I want to thank my family: my husband and son who courageously assist me in my everyday academic work. I dedicate this book to both of you.

Introduction

The movie *127 hours*[1] is about an energetic and joyful man in his twenties, obsessed with canyoning and biking escapades. At the start of a lone excursion aimed at breaking a mountain biking record, he sets his watch—which from then on will count the time of the journey—and races through the canyon while narrating his journey to the camera mounted on his bike's handlebars. Despite being surrounded by breathtaking views and nature, he isolates himself from his immediate environment by putting on headphones and listening to loud music. In pursuit of his record-breaking feat, his bike breaks down and he is forced to complete his journey on foot. Suddenly, he falls into the precipice and a large rock follows him, crushing his hand and blocking his way out.

The young man spends 127 hours trapped in the canyon while documenting his struggle to survive in a series of video recordings. The full realization of his precarious position and the possibility of death prompts him to look for a solution. The contents of his backpack, including a sports watch, a video camera, a head-mounted mirror, and a music player reveal that he possesses almost no practical tools that could be of use, i.e., a penknife that the hero had left at home. Not having a smartphone might seem astonishing, but this could be due to the lack of reception in the desert; it is the electronic technology that seems to be indispensable. It accompanies the man both during the gripping adventure and in the moment of his near-death. Finally, the hero—acutely aware of the possibility of the inevitable end—amputates his arm with a blunt tool to free himself. By causing himself unimaginable pain, he saves his life, but before he leaves the precipice . . . he takes a photo of his arm trapped by the rock, still dripping with blood.

This story—based on real-life events—illustrates the paradoxes caused by mediatization. Physical activity, exercise, sport, and recreation, are technologized and subjected to the process of mediatization. They are transformed into hybrid clusters of practices that simultaneously isolate us and connect us to different aspects of life. A music player isolates the listener from his immediate environment, from the sounds of wild nature, but it integrates him with the physically remote—yet emotionally close—world of stimulating music. A watch allows to monitor and control time, but it takes away freedom of timelessness, affecting the pace of a journey, which, in the example above, is supposed to end up with breaking a record. The video his camera records and the photos it takes prevent the protagonist of the story to be "in the moment" because he focuses on documenting the present for the future. In addition, the video-taping equipment becomes a necessary tool to record and persevere the grisly moments of his deathly ordeal with the hope of someone learning about it one day.

Media technology turns out to be more important than practical tools, even though the latter are necessary to survive in extreme conditions. A camera or a music player at hand . . . are not objects thanks to which anger can be released, when something essential is missing . . . that is water; when there is no sharp knife at hand, but there is a flashing video camera light. It does not bear frustration . . . because media technology has become a natural companion, technology that is close, obvious, explicit, and for that reason, invisible—or visible only in specific circumstances. In addition, it gives one a chance to interact with oneself and can be a means offering comfort or hope.

Media technology in the processual dimension, i.e., technology in practice, exhibits a paradoxical nature since, despite its obvious physical dimension, it is characterized by a peculiar transparency. Just as clothes are obvious, and thus unnoticeable objects to which people pay attention in particular contexts, they are accepted as a norm, an ever-present and thus invisible aspect of one's daily life. Therefore, one does not regret having packed a shirt and trousers, yet not enough water, since clothes are indisputable and almost imperceptible objects to carry. Similarly, the physical load of the backpack heavy with electronic equipment is no longer a ballast, but a natural need, even a necessity. It seems that one cannot do without media technologies. The processual and material properties of technologies are becoming indispensable for the users who are willing to compromise their comfort and, as in the case of the aforementioned here, their chances of survival for the price of the benefits media technologies offer.

Two antithetical trends are worth noticing in that context. On the one hand, it is evident that everyday life exposed and saturated by surrounding technology and mediating devices, invariably transforms. This is fostered by relatively universal access to technology, its ever-diverging offer resulting in penetration into and integration with almost every area of human life. Subsequently, it leads to deepening mediatization on both individual and social levels. On the other hand, it can reach a degree of over-saturation that stimulates a retreat; this is when certain properties and processes become a burden to their recipients. In other words, losses begin to dominate over benefits and, as a consequence, technologies begin to lose their dominance and become viewed as unnecessary. Users give them up, and the activities they undertake begin to acquire a more analogue nature. The number of technology present in some aspects of life decreases, both in quantitative and qualitative dimensions. This leads to desaturation, although the world around it remains mediatized.

The goal of this book is to depict the complexity of mediatization mechanisms resulting from the presence and use of media technologies. Focusing on physical activity, it aims to determine the characteristics of the mediatization process: what technology properties and what attributes of processes mediated by technology lead to physical activity mediatization. It will also examine what causes the reverse tendencies to arise. This study focuses on physically active users of technology who are subjected to mediatization and examines the process's mechanisms on both individual and social level. Widespread presence, deep infiltration, and numerous consequences of intensive media technology use is observed. Media saturation serves here as a quantitative and qualitative research parameter. Thus, the book also offers a new methodological proposal. It presents the results of surveys used as a test of the research procedure through the integration of the quantitative and qualitative dimensions. By deploying surveys, analyses, and statistical calculations, individual interviews and observations, it proposes the use of an original measurement tool in the study of mediatization of everyday life, which enables quantification and a deeper exploration of the phenomenon. According to Friedrich Krotz, the essence of research on mediatization lies in studying of the presence of new media technologies in everyday life, their integration with ordinary practices and the following consequences since people "communicate and *act* (emphasis in the original) differently on the basis of these newly introduced media."[2] This book explains not only the mediatizing qualities and power of communication, but also examines other processes, unrestricted to communication, yet deriving from the use of media technologies.

Based on metatheoretical studies and empirical quantitative and qualitative studies of physical activity, two dimensions of the media saturation parameter were determined: the quality of saturation and the quantity of saturation. The first property corresponds with the practical aspects of media technologies, i.e., through its functions, affordances, mechanisms of operation, and usage techniques. The second one refers to the intensity of media presence and use, and positions it within its quantitative dimension by the ratio of the saturation spectrum and saturation degree.

The conducted research allowed to determine the mechanisms of mediatization and the consequences of the extensive presence of media technologies in users' lives. Alongside the dynamic development of new media technologies and their application across a vast range of areas, mediatization is becoming a much wider and a more complex phenomenon, encompassing not only the problems of information transmission and reception but also of the material and physical aspects of technology usage, including but not limited to content creation, distribution, and consumption. The conceptualization based on metatheoretical[3] studies, allows for the formulation of definitions and typologies, and the subsequent testing and the development of the theoretical framework of media saturation parameter. This, in turn, allows for the examination of the extent to which the world of physical activity is saturated by the media and the exploration of mediatization mechanisms.

THE CORE CONCEPTS: INTERACTIVE COMMUNICATION AND MEDIA TECHNOLOGIES

Moving away from the basic form of face-to-face communication, Fredrich Krotz distinguishes three main types of communication through the media: mediated interpersonal communication, communication with standardized, widely addressed content (formerly called mass media content), and interactive communication.[4] The last type of communication has a particularly significant effect on mediatization of physical activity. This is due to the growing importance of mobile technologies that serve as a defining factor impacting the direction and quality of the communication transformation. Devices, particularly mobile accessories, dominate physical activity, and to a large extent they neither facilitate interpersonal communication nor communication with standardized content. It is a type of communication in which "there must not be another human person involved."[5] F. Krotz also indicates the fourth type of communication: passive communication, which he further divides into intended and unintended communication.[6] Passive communication takes place when users are the subject of communication (e.g., when their data is analyzed by search engines). Both passive and interactive communication as well as their hybrids facilitate mediatization of physical activity.

The importance of interactive and passive communication is grounded in the transformative power of digital technologies in users' everyday life. In this context, it is becoming more important to explore the specifics of media change, and to a lesser extent, the change in communication. John Postill, referring to the example of studies on mobile media use in China, considers legitimacy of the idea that media devices that are not only used as "communication devices," but to, i.e., listening to a recording, "should be brought under the umbrella of communication?"[7] We observe "transition from communicativity to mediality."[8] There is a need to answer the question of how to examine and interpret the media; in other words—how to understand media technologies.

According to Mark Hansen, we have "the opportunity to explore the 'transduction' of message and media that [. . .] becomes generalized in our contemporary media age. Transduction, following Gilbert Simondon's conceptualization, is a relation in which the relation itself holds primacy over the terms related."[9] Tranduction in media definition allows us to take a holistic view and look at the structure of relations. Because in such an approach, the structure of relations is more important than the elements connected with this relation. Media can be perceived as "environment for life"[10]—all media are something in between; they are what mediates,[11] what "is implicated in the living as essentially technical."[12] In this sense, media—an intrinsically technical environment—define living conditions and "human technogenesis,"[13] reciprocal human and technical evolution where "human and media development are intertwined in a helixlike embrace."[14] Raymond Williams, described media as "technology and cultural form"[15]—combining both, seemingly differing aspects. From a broad perspective, media are a kind of technology—media technology, which serves as an intermediary between different elements. It is worth noting that technology can mediate both: communication between human beings and the use of data and information by a single individual (interactive communication). In this context, mediation, which examines the process of using data and information, plays a key role in the era of digitization. David Hakken, discussing information and communication as "digitally-mediated human activity,"[16] points out that it is increasingly more difficult to distinguish one from the other. That does not change the fact that in some activities the second person is present (making it an explicit interpersonal communication activity), and in others it is not (a communication activity between a person and technology). The term "new media" was introduced to distinguish the actual breakthrough that took place in the evolution[17] seen as the new phase of techno-genesis, which has been determined not so much by specific technological artefacts as by their technical capacities.[18] The importance of new media, or rather modern media technologies, is based not only on their properties (although due to their specificity and range of mediated processes they co-decide on mediatization), but on a deeper evolutionary change, which is determined by the growing importance of media usage not only in relation to communication through the media in classic (interpersonal) understanding. The importance of exchanging information is growing, including the raw, unprocessed data between people and devices, and the broad system in which no other receiver participates directly. Mediatization is therefore based on two channels: communication and media usage.

Using the media can stand for communication (one-to-one, one-to-many, many-to-many, etc.), and, in some cases, communication occurs in a highly mediated manner (e.g., with the device designer, through interaction with the product of their vision and its technological functionalities).[19] Above all, however, its digital aspect cannot be overlooked since it leads to a new, extra-communicational way of using media since "media, nowadays, are no longer simply means of communication but at the same time and additionally are means of collecting data about us as their users in real time."[20] This highlights the concept of "datafication"[21] where

> "media are not *only* (emphasis in original) means of technologically based communication any more. (. . .) Processes of social construction through media no longer refer only to human communication, but also to the automatized accumulation and calculation of the data we produce while we use digital devices for communication."[22]

Thus, the scope of media technologies is not limited to infrastructure, devices, software, services, or their integrated complexes enabling personal communication, but it embodies a resource with which individuals interact (through the physical and digital interface) and exchange data and information—in F. Krotz's words: communicate interactively. Thus we can observe the distinction between the use of media and the use of communication, also in the context of the question about media related change.[23]

Modern digital media technologies are characterized by a specific nature. The media is based on big data: creating, storing, processing, and the flow of ever-growing amount of data. Therefore, it is possible to distinguish between *communicative media technologies* as well as *data and information media technologies*. Within the complex context of media and technology relationship, the media can be thus seen "as technologies and sign structures."[24] Media technologies serve therefore as a tool, a machinery which includes specific content which—when integrated—implicates specific practices.

> "(. . .) technology is, on the one hand, an identifiable, relatively durable entity, a physically, economically, politically, and socially organized phenomenon in space-time. It has material and cultural properties that transcend the experience of individuals and particular settings. In this aspect, it is what we may call a technological artifact, which appears in our lives as a specific machine, technique, appliance, device, or gadget. At the same time, use of the technology involves a repeatedly experienced, personally ordered and edited version of the technological artifact, being experienced differently by different individuals and differently by the same individuals depending on the time or circumstance."[25]

Based on numerous functions and mechanisms of operation, technology enables the exchange of data and information that serve other activities.

In addition, due to diversity of mediatization definitions, approaches, and paradigms within which mediatization is examined, it seems more appropriate to refer to the category of media technologies, rather than media or new media, which makes it possible to explain the essence of the mechanisms of mediatization. F. Krotz believes that only when technology is used for communication purposes, it becomes a medium;[26] a term traditionally reserved for interpersonal communication (regardless of the scale, level, and scope). Meanwhile, the term media technologies exceeds that interpersonal dimension. It puts emphasis on technology, which takes on mediating character, encompassing interpersonal and beyond interpersonal exchange. Additionally, in the media ecology tradition, technology takes on an integrated character. It constitutes of infrastructure, devices, software, data, and information complexities.[27] In summary, media technologies are technical tools by means of which users communicate (regardless of the dimension and nature of communication) and/or by means of which they manage data and information. Nowadays, these are mainly digital technologies, although this does not mean that analogue technologies, even those traditional ones, including a paper notebook and a pen, are not used in physical activity. However, their impact is negligible.

THEORETICAL AND METHODOLOGICAL CHALLENGES

In accordance with the adopted perspective, media technologies are tools that mediate contact with data and information, and modify and transform various spheres of human life. Media technologies transform lives in a structural and processual sense, because they are instruments of action. They are symbolic, aesthetic, material, and functional[28] objects that find practical applications in everyday life. Both at the individual and societal level, and at their intersection, various transformations take place, which are best illustrated by mediatized physical activity. Interactive and passive communication determine the course of physical activity modification to an increasing degree: both in the mental and physical dimensions, and especially on the border between the two spheres into which media technologies enter with their structure and the potential to implement specific processes.

Theory

"The central question related to mediatization is how to study it empirically and to grasp it theoretically. A key element for understanding is to ask how people introduce new media technologies into their everyday lives, how they appropriate these media and integrate them into their lives, and what consequences will arise from that, as they communicate and act differently on the basis of these newly introduced media."[29]

Thus, studying mediatization requires determining the course of three phases: the introduction of media to in a specific environment, their entrenchment in everyday life, and the subsequent implications. It is based on the analysis of "a lot of single mechanisms and dependencies in detail,"[30] the examination of "transforming direction or tendency."[31] This is done both at the micro (individual) level and at the mezzo (collective) level. Within the context of this study, this applies to the representatives of specific sports disciplines (or in a broader sense: particular forms physical activity) and formations of this disciplines and collectivities built around them.

In this study mediatization is observed "from *below*: changing the lives of individuals in their immediate environments,"[32] considering the material properties of media technologies and the micro-dynamics of processes carried out by the individual.

"We need to understand technology, especially our media and information technologies in just such a context if we are to grasp the subtleties, power and consequences of technological change. For technologies are social things, suffused with the symbolic, and vulnerable to the eternal paradoxes and contradictions of social life, both in their creation and in their use. The study of the media, I maintain, in turn requires such a questioning of technology."[33]

Recognizing the subtleties and paradoxes, which Roger Silverstone encouraged many years ago, it is not focused on mediatization as such, but mediatization of a concrete area; in particular "lifeworld."[34]

This leads to the question of how the actual operationalization of concepts and theories should be carried out in concrete empirical studies.[35] After adopting particular terminological and definitional assumptions, one should adopt an approach that allows to examine the versatility and complexity of the relationship between media technologies and everyday life, as well as the changeable nature of these relationships deriving from the fact that the media are transformed from those that accompany life into a fundamental experience. As a result of media intrusion, the environment becomes "media-soaked,"[36] and subsequently media become neutral and, with time, even "invisible" like "epistemic wallpapers."[37] Researching mediatization, therefore, requires a thorough examination of "interlocking technical, social, and biological processes of mediation."[38]

The adopted perspective should also respond to the challenges posed to the researchers of mediatization, including the development of:

- "more middle-range explorations,"[39]
- "additional concepts at lower levels of abstraction,"[40]
- "further concepts and approaches to describe *in detail* (emphasis in original) how the transformation that we relate to the term mediatization actually takes place,"[41]
- noticing elements common to various theories, traditions, and paradigms, "focus on what unites different approaches to media and change (mediatization, mediation, polymedia, medium theory, etc.), a task that has sometimes been neglected."[42]

An additional challenge derives from the necessity to identify and analyze what is there to the research procedure (saturation), but also what is not there (desaturation),[43] in line with David Hakken's recommendations:

"first: identifying social changes, or the absence thereof, that correlate with digital mediation. With regard to evident change correlates, one should then consider how frequently a change is present with a particular mediation and how frequently it is absent, as well as trying to grasp to range of its relevant possible forms."[44]

Reflecting on the importance of media technologies must therefore go beyond the rigid framework of social sciences. Having a transdisciplinary character, it should be located at the crossroads of the humanities, social, natural, and technical sciences to capture the mechanisms of mediatization. A comprehensive understanding of the transformations taking place in the life of modern media technology users is possible only by adapting a cross-disciplinary perspective encompassing sociological, psychological, technical, media, and culture studies. In other words, it requires the use of diverse and integrated application of research tools.

Methodology

In the presented study, a mixed approach was applied that is characterized by collecting different types of data to draw a comprehensive picture of the examined problem. The study began with a survey carried out within a specific population: young, physically active individuals, living in large European urban agglomeration (Wroclaw, Poland), declared using media technologies during physical activity. In the second phase, qualitative research using

interviews, observations, and content analysis was conducted to gather detailed insight. John Creswell postulates that the mixed approach should rely
on the use of sequential strategies; therefore the data was first collected in
phases and then integrated by merging and embedding to ensure efficient use
of tools necessary to investigate such complex processes.[45]

Additionally and to aid that goal, indirect data collected during the first
phase was mixed with the second phase data. This included merging and embedding quantitative and qualitative data between different collection stages
as well as during the process of its interpretation when the qualitative data
was partially immersed in quantitative data.

The methods deployed in the second phase were aimed to answer a different set of research questions than those used in the first phase of the
project. In the first stage, the aim was to investigate the scope and spectrum
of media saturation and the perception of individual elements of media usage by the respondents. The second stage analysis focused on the individual
participant level, examining why and how mediatization occurs by taking
into account technological and processual dimension of media saturation
and its implications for the individual and collective level. The data obtained in both stages was integrated in order to analyze mediatization using
media saturation as its key parameter.

The adopted strategy is therefore of a sequential explanatory nature: the
quantitative data from the first phase of research served as a basis for qualitative research conducted in the second phase.[46] The explanatory strategy is
particularly effective when seeking to clarify and interpret dependencies.[47] In
the first stage, a numerical description of tendencies and opinions explored by
a survey were sought[48] while the second stage allowed for a deeper exploration of the phenomenon based on the integrated instrumentation of qualitative
research methods.

Two main stages were selected for the implemented project: quantitative
surveys with the use of a questionnaire and qualitative research with the use
of integrated tools. Depending on a particular phase of the second stage, semi-
structured, in-depth interviews supplemented with the original photographic
material and a case study integrating interviews, observation, and analysis of
individually collected data (photographs, films, and statistics coming from
mobile applications) were deployed. When examining the use of embedded
model applied on several levels of analysis,[49] the descent from the level of the
studied population to its individual representatives was applied.

The analysis of qualitative data was based on recommendations applied in
grounded theory research and a case study methodology. The coding was applied utilizing the following codes: situation and contexts, attitudes of the participants, thinking patterns, processes and activities.[50] Through the application

of the codes, theoretical models explaining the qualitative aspects of media saturation and enabling "understanding how things occur" were constructed.[51]

During the stage of qualitative research, as well as in the final stage of integration of the results, a holistic approach toward the interpretation was used to "develop a complex picture of the problem or issue under study. This implies reporting multiple perspectives, identifying the many factors involved in a situation and generally sketching the larger picture that emerges."[52] In addition, data analysis focused on the problem of complementing the methodological and methodical aspects of mediatization theory with the media saturation parameter, providing the interpretation with data acquired from a specific area (physical activity).

CHAPTER CONTENT

Chapter 1 establishes the concept of media saturation and the methods of examining it. It demonstrates that the roots of the concept lie in materialist phenomenology and media ecology (including medium theory). Also, it outlines a definite relationship with theory of mediatization and justifies the introduction and operationalization of the concept of saturation as a response to the challenges that research into this area poses. The chapter provides an answer to the following question: how does mediatization happen? It accentuates the importance of a social and individual technology-user relationship in researching mediatization. The chapter presents meta-theoretical analyses that lead to a definition of media saturation. It explains why abductive reasoning has been deployed for the purpose of the study. Based on the methodological assumptions of studies on mediatization, it illustrates the course in which subject theory is deducted from metatheory, which in turn further serves the development of metatheory. In addition, the chapter examines media studies literature representing diverse definitions of saturation and the perspectives adapted to research it outside of the mediatization studies while providing arguments supporting a new take on the problem. The last part of the chapter defines saturation as a key parameter of mediatization. It describes technological (structural) and processual saturation in detail while specifying its quantitative and qualitative components that allow to identify mediatization mechanisms, both on the individual and social level. Finally, a rationale is provided as to why it is necessary to examine desaturation and the potential demediatization of particular areas of everyday life. The chapter concludes with the justification of the choice of amateur physical activity and the sport-media worlds as a valid and appropriate area serving as an empirical test case of the media saturation parameter in mediatization research.

Chapter 2 characterizes the sample population (15–24 years old, living in urban area—Wroclaw agglomeration, Poland) and the survey sample in detail. It presents survey results including: basic preferred forms of activity, media technologies used (the spectrum of technologies), mediated processes that take place (the spectrum of processes), and advanced measurements of the variants of degrees of technological saturation. The chapter presents survey results on qualitative properties of technological saturation (the importance of particular technologies, their functions, and implications: influence on the activity, physical condition, health and appearance) and also on processual saturation (mainly the importance of interpersonal communication during physical activity).

Chapter 3 includes results of qualitative technological saturation to research (properties of audio technologies, multifunctional technologies, and sport self-trackers) as well as processual saturation (properties and flow of the listening processes, communication and self-tracking). It illustrates interpretations which lead to the identification of mediatization mechanisms on the micro level.

Chapter 4 justifies the choice for qualitative research (an individual, in-depth semi-structured interviews, and video recorded observations) of respondents who get engaged in niche forms of physical activity defined in the survey (cross-fit, calisthenics, silhouette fitness, paragliding, skiing, rowing, horse riding, western-style horse riding, parkour, dancing, pole dance, MMA, figure roller-skating) and who deploy comparatively niche technologies identified in the survey (stand-alone digital cameras and digital cameras in smartphones). This chapter presents results on the qualitative technological saturation specifics (properties of video recording technologies) and processes mediated through video recording (analysis; memorializing; communication; self-presentation and promotion). It includes interpretations that lead to specifying concrete mechanisms of mediatization on the micro- and mezzo-level.

Chapter 5 includes justification of the research on desaturation that arises from theoretical presumptions and the qualitative research results carried out in earlier stages of the research. It presents desaturation research results performed through individual in-depth semi-structured interviews, among participants who have resigned from using technologies or who have never adopted them during physical activity. The chapter includes the description of characteristics pertaining to absolute and relative desaturation and models of desaturating users. It is concluded by the specification of technologies that are most often rejected by the users (self-trackers, music players).

The final chapter integrates a vast array of research results. It illustrates bilateral relations between media technologies and physical activity. It describes general impact of physical activity on media technology usage resulting in its universalization, integration of media technologies into other everyday activities, indirect expectations of users in relation to media technology design, functionalities, and accessories, to mention just a few. The chapter explains and elaborates on the impact of media technology on physical activity: modulation of physical activity (on micro level), transformation of sport disciplines (on mezzo level), hybridization of physical and everyday activities, and the emergence of desaturation. The last section presents the conclusions drawn from the applied methods and research tools, the potential and possibilities for the development of the methodology are indicated. The book concludes with a justification of the applicability of the concept in the research of other areas of everyday life.

NOTES

1. *127 Hours*, directed by Danny Boyle (2010; London: 20th Century Fox Home Entertainment, 2011), DVD.
2. Friedrich Krotz, "From a Social Worlds Perspective to the Analysis of Mediatized Worlds," in: *Media Practice and Everyday Agency in Europe*, eds. Leif Kramp Leif Kramp, Nico Carpentier, Andreas Hepp, Ilija Tomanić Trivundža, Hannu Nieminen, Risto Kunelius, Tobias Olsson, Ebba Sundin and Richard Kilborn (Bremen: Edition Lumière, 2014), 73.
3. Metatheories are "general theoretical constructs resting in part upon empirical evidence, but which are not empirically verifiable in their entirety," in: Andreas Hepp, *Cultures of Mediatization* (Cambridge, MA: Polity, 2013), 49.
4. Friedrich Krotz, "Media as a Societal Structure and a Situational Frame for Communicative Action: A Definition of Concepts," in: *Critical Perspectives on the European Mediasphere*, eds. Ilija Tomanić Trivundža, Nico Carpentier, Hannu Nieminen, Pille Pruulmann-Venerfeldt, Richard Kilborn, Ebba Sundin and Tobias Olsson (Lubljana: Faculty of Social Sciences: Založba FDV, 2011): 36.
5. Friedrich Krotz and Andreas Hepp, "A Concretization of Mediatization: How 'Mediatization Works' and Why Mediatized Worlds are a Helpful Concept for Empirical Mediatization Research," *Empedocles: European Journal for the Philosophy of Communication* 3.2 (2011): 142.
6. Krotz, "Media as a Societal Structure . . ." 37.
7. John Postill and Brian Larkin, "Theorising Media and Change" (e-seminar, Melbourne, December 5–19), Media Anthropology Network European Association of Social Anthropologists (EASA) E-Seminar Series (2003), 28 (retrieved online).
8. Siegfried J. Schmidt, "Media Philosophy—A Reasonable Programme?" in *Philosophy of the Information Society. 30th Wittgenstein Symposium* (Frankfurt u. a.: Ontos, 2007), 95 (retrieved online).
9. Simondon, Gilbert, *Du Mode des Objects Techniques* (Paris: Aubier, 1989) quoted in Mark, B. Hansen, "Media Theory" *Theory, Culture & Society* 23 (2–3) (2006): 300.

10. Ibid., 299.

11. Hansen refers to the Latin meaning of the term medium prior to its inclusion in English language dictionary: "meaning middle, center, midst, intermediated course, thus something implying mediation or an intermediary," ibid., 300.

12. Ibid., 300. Although Kember and Zylinska are inclined toward understanding mediation as remediation, they also treat media as "particular enactments of *tekhnē* (emphasis in original) or as temporal "fixings" of technological and other forms of becoming," Sarah Kember and Joanna Zylinska, *Life After New Media: Mediation as a Vital Process* (Cambridge, MA: MIT Press, 2012), 21.

13. Hansen, ibid., 301.

14. Gary Gumpert and Robert Cathcart, "A Theory of Mediation," in: *Mediation, Information and Communication*, ed. Brent D. Ruben and Leah A. Lievrouw (New Brunswick, NJ: Transaction, 1990), 35.

15. Raymond Williams, *Television: Technology and Cultural Form* (London: Routledge, 1990).

16. Davin Hakken, e-seminar post from December 12, 2013 in: Postill and Larkin, ibid.

17. Gumpert and Cathcart, ibid., 35.

18. Mark, B. Hansen, ibid., 304–05.

19. Andrew Dewdney and Peter Ride, *The Digital Media Handbook* (London: Routledge, 2013), 112.

20. Andreas Hepp and Uwe Hasebrink, "Researching Transforming Communications in Times of Deep Mediatization: A Figurational Approach," in: *Communicative Figurations, Transforming Communications—Studies in Cross-Media Research*, ed. Andreas Hepp, Andreas Breiter, Uwe Hasebrink (Cham: Palgrave McMillan, 2016): 16.

21. José Van Dijck, "Datafication, Dataism and Dataveillance: Big Data between Scientific Paradigm and Ideology," *Surveillance & Society* 12.2 (2014): 197.

22. Andreas Hepp, Andreas Breiter, and Uwe Hasebrink, "Rethinking Transforming Communication: An Introduction," in: *Communicative Figurations, Transforming Communications—Studies in Cross-Media Research*, ed. Andreas Hepp, Andreas Breiter, Uwe Hasebrink (Cham: Palgrave McMillan, 2016): 5–6.

23. Aeron Davis, *The Mediation of Power: A Critical Introduction* (London: Routledge, 2007), 13.

24. Göran Bolin, "The Rhythm of Ages: Analyzing Mediatization Through the Lens of Generations across Cultures," *International Journal of Communication* 10 (2016): 5253.

25. Wanda Orlikowski, "Using Technology and Constituting Structures: A Practice Lens for Studying Technology in Organisations," *Organisation Science*, 11 (4) (2000): 408.

26. Krotz, "Media as a Societal Structure . . ." 33.

27. In literature, other terms are also present, such as "digital and computational technology," e.g. Marian T. Adolf and Nico Stehr, "The Return of Social Physics?" in *The Technology of Information, Communication and Administration—An Entwined History* (Bern: Swiss Federal Archives, 2015), 3 (retrieved online). Sport and physical

activity researchers use the term "media technologies" adopted also here; sometimes the term "digital media technologies" is also used, e.g., Clifton Evers, "Researching Action Sport with a GoPro TM Camera: An Embodied and Emotional Mobile Video Tale of the Sea, Masculinity and Men-who-surf," in: *Researching Embodied Sport: Exploring Movement Cultures. Routledge Research in Sport, Culture and Society*, ed. Ian Wellard (London: Routlede, 2015).

28. Roger Silverstone and Leslie Haddon, "Design and the Domestication of Information and Communication Technologies: Technical Change and Everyday Life," in: *Communication by Design: The Politics of Information and Communication Technologies*, ed. Robin Mansell and Roger Silverstone (Oxford, UK: Oxford University Press, 1996): 44.

29. Krotz, "From a Social Worlds . . ." 73.

30. Friedrich Krotz, "Explaining the Mediatisation Approach" *Javnost-The Public* 24.2 (2017): 109.

31. Knut Lundby, "Mediatization of Communication," in: *Mediatization of Communication*, ed. Knut Lundby (Boston: De Guyter, 2014), 23.

32. Ibid., 23.

33. Roger Silverstone, *Why Study the Media?* (London: Sage Reference, 1999): 8. doi: http://dx.doi.org/10.4135/9781446219461.

34. Hepp and Krotz, ibid., 11.

35. Which, according to K. Lundby, is significantly harder than the discussion about general theory. Lundby, ibid., 21.

36. Todd Gitlin, "Supersaturation, or, the Media Torrent and Disposable Feeling," in: *Living in the Information Age,* ed. Erik P. Bucy (Belmond: Wadsworth Thomson, 2005): 142.

37. Nigel Thrift. "Movement-space: the Changing Domain of Thinking Resulting from the Development of New Kinds of Spatial Awareness," *Economy and Society* 33(4) (2004): 585.

38. Kember and Zylinska, ibid., p. 140.

39. Kirsten Drotner, "Boundaries and Bridges: Digital Storytelling in Education Studies and Media Studies," in: *Digital Storytelling, Mediatized Stories*, ed. Knut Lundby (New York: Peter Lang 2008): 61–81.

40. David Deacon and James Stanyer, "Mediatization: Key Concept or Conceptual Bandwagon?" *Media, Culture & Society* 36.7 (2014): 12.

41. Hepp and Hasebrink, ibid., 18.

42. Emiliano Treré's e-seminar post from December 10, 2013, in Postill and Larkin, ibid., 20.

43. E.g., "the abandonment of 'new' media networks and technologies should interest mediatization scholars just as greatly as their adoption," David Deacon and James Stanyer, ibid.,10.

44. Davin Hakken, e-seminar post from December 12, 2013 in Postill and Larkin, ibid., 26.

45. Michael D. Fetters, Leslie A. Curry, and John W. Creswell, "Achieving Integration in Mixed Methods Designs—Principles and Practices," *Health Services Research* 48 (2013).

46. John W. Creswell, *Research Design: Qualitative, Quantitative, and Mixed Methods Approaches* (Los Angeles: Sage Publications, 2009), 211.

47. Ibid., 211.

48. Ibid., 145.

49. Ibid., 219.

50. Ibid., 187.

51. Ibid., 195.

52. Ibid., 176.

Chapter One

Theory of Media Saturation

THEORETICAL AND META-THEORETICAL FOUNDATIONS OF MEDIA SATURATION

The concepts presented in this book are based on the methodological assumption gravitating toward oscillation between the materialist and phenomenological dimension of the media,[1] integration of research on media, and communication of its materialist and symbolic (virtual) dimension.[2] Obliterating the media division into empirical and transcendental dimensions allows for capturing in a comprehensive, interdisciplinary, and balanced way both "experiential dimensions of media" and "technical logics of media,"[3] which play equally important roles in the mediatization process. In this context and in reference to Marshall McLuhan's concepts (the famous "medium is the message"[4]), Mark Hansen explains how the change in the definition of media allowed for extending of the hermeneutic analyses by physical and technical elements.[5] From a transduction perspective, the relationship between content and technology is more important than the elements that are related to each other: content itself and technology itself. Similarly, the relationship between technology and culture is more important than those two spheres themselves.[6] Analyzing that relationship has since become more important than studying isolated media elements, especially the content. The foundations for the development of the media saturation concept presented here are both of hermeneutic and materialist nature, with the latter attempted to be situated within materialist phenomenology when appropriate. This, in turn, requires to be complemented with an ecological perspective—a return to the roots in research on the transduction of media technology and culture.

Materialist Phenomenology and Media Ecology

A slightly modified version of the materialist phenomenology by Andreas Hepp and Nick Couldry, complemented with the concept of the media environment developed within media ecology, and a proposition of a new parameter for studying media saturation has been adopted as a methodological basis for the presented analyses.

One of the assumptions of the phenomenological-materialist approach by N. Couldry and A. Hepp states that "the social is constructed from, and through, technologically mediated processes and infrastructures of communication, that is, through what we have come to call 'media.'"[7] The media, thus, encompasses "contents and infrastructure derived from institutionally sustained technologies of communication."[8] The proposed theoretical perspective puts a distinct emphasis on the physical infrastructure of communication[9] since mediation is based on technology.[10] Both the immaterial (semantic) and the physical (infrastructural) dimension of communication processes play key roles in constructing social reality.

Although the proposal of N. Couldry and A. Hepp integrates both dimensions in the study of mediatization, it remains at a relatively high level of generalization and is rather limited to the importance of technology in the processes of institutionalization that takes place at three levels: self-organization in media practice; forms and patterns of communicating through the media; and media organizations.[11] The authors mention the importance of affordances, infrastructure, and devices, but they do not elaborate on their significance and role, which seem crucial to determine how mediatization occurs, in order not to limit ourselves to the effects, but examine the specificity of transformation, as e.g., A. Hepp writes.[12] Mediatization takes place not only due to the communication of content and its subsequent construction of social meaning and emergence of other collective processes, but also as a result of practical application of technology and its individual consequences, including the creation of purely individual, personal relationships with the media that serve as a key foundation for the micro-management of one's activities.

In order to include the individual perspectives and aspects of mediatization within the scope of the analysis and thus persevere the significance of the phenomenon at its micro level, it is proposed to adopt a perspective located at the crossroad of materialistic phenomenology and traditional media ecology, which integrates social and individual, materialist and symbolic dimensions.

Communication by media technologies, and even more so, communication with media technologies,[13] allows for shaping the reality through their use. This applies to constructing the reality of one's own personal relations with the media, as well as constructing the reality of the social, shared media world. A media technology user creates his own constellations of platforms and networks of practices, without the need for sharing them with other users. Broadly understood interactive and passive communication takes place between individuals and devices, their multiple extensions, platforms, data, and systems that define the confines and possibilities of actions. Therefore, not only can it be defined as a set of consequences of "infrastructure of mediated communication"[14] for social communication, but also as the result of interactions of an individual with a device on the mental and physical level, creating a complex infrastructure where "modes of action are enframed by these technologies."[15] Undoubtedly, communication, or, in a broader sense, interaction with the technology, also possesses the characteristics of strongly mediated social communication. Each device has been designed by an individual and communication with it in a highly mediated manner can be classified as a type of communication with its designer, e.g., a mobile application used in a daily activity communicates through its interface and its functionalities a particular vision of activity formulated by the designer. However, while this aspect of communication deserves attention, the user-device relationship remains a central factor contributing to mediatization.

The second area requiring internal integration is—as discussed in the Introduction—a separation of communication and use that underlies the proposed definition of media technology. Paraphrasing Roger Silverstone's stance that the "object dimension" is as important as the "content dimension,"[16] it can be said that the communication (of the content) is as important as the use (of the object). This translates into the necessity to go beyond linguistic pragmatism or broadly understood communication (regardless of the level, scale, and scope) in the analysis of mediatization. It occurs due to the interaction of users with technology, mainly with devices and information systems collecting and managing huge resources of data. This intricate process is further complicated by ubiquitous computing obscuring the distinction between interactions among users from the interaction of users with technologies.[17] From a sociological perspective, it embodies a wider problem of artificial separation of social communication and communication with technology while eliminating seemingly noncommunication technologies, i.e., technologies that do not serve interpersonal communication, even mass communication but are strongly associated with the network of other technologies, and indirectly with networks of users. Media technologies that mediatize reality include both those facilitating communication between users as well as those not serving interpersonal interaction but positioned in a dense network of technology and user relationships, and hence involved in the process of social communication in a heavily mediated manner.

The materialistic dimension of phenomenology must take into account the complex nature of communication, technology and, consequently, their materiality. On the one hand, media technologies are artifacts, and on the other, they are technology-in-practice.[18] In addition, they exhibit their properties and functions in a defined context. Technologies as artifacts assume physicality, tangibility of "objects." They are objects, but display their properties through performativity.[19] Therefore, we could determine this materiality as factual or artifactual. The resource of all features, properties, and affordances is hidden within. The analysis of artifactual materiality allows to define the essence of technology, and due to its structures, identify its functions which generate certain consequences.

This approach is close to the proposal of Niels Ole Finnemann, who postulates a departure from "media logic" in favor of "media grammar," which consists of "enabling and disabling capacities, the constraints, affordances, and biases of various media and media constellations."[20] In media properties, especially in new media, the author sees evident conditioning for mediatization. Focusing on the properties of technology leads to an understanding of the core of the deep media change processes, at the macro, mezzo, and micro level, i.e., when the media is woven into daily activities.[21]

Since everyday life is shaped by both protocols and the use of media,[22] its change is only possible through technology-in-use.[23] In this context, materiality must also be understood as "ability to instantiate ideas in practice"[24] and the means of its application is key. As Paul Leonardi points out, not every feature, not every use is as important as the others, so technology is not always material in character. Media materiality reveals itself via properties that are important for the user, "so researchers should ask, when examining practices of use, which features are 'material' (significant) for this user and how those features become significant for the type of work she does, for whom she interact with, or for maintaining control."[25] In this context, it is not important whether the artifact is physical or digital;[26] but how technology was used. In practice, thus, the constellations of technologies created by users are of a hybrid nature, encompassing both their physical and digital characteristics.

In the context of materiality and artefactual nature of media technologies, it seems justifiable to supplement the perspective of materialistic phenomenology with the achievements of the medium theory, or, more broadly, with media ecology. Both perspectives have always been closely related, and in the context of the development of the theory of mediatization, media ecology poses a great potential for furthering the understanding of mediatization. According to Lynn Schofield Clark, it is the theory of the medium that may allow mediatization researchers to go a step further, i.e., "to develop not only coherence, but also diagnosis."[27] This requires considering related and increasingly convergent media as an environment[28] and studying "their structure, content, and impact on people."[29] Going beyond the perspective of a specific environment of one chosen medium is what Johua Meyrowitz emphasizes.[30] Andreas Hepp, Andreas Breiter, and Uwe Hasebrink specify "a cross media approach" as looking from the perspective of integrated environment—"analysis how the various media come together in the communicative construction of social domains."[31] Lance Strate states: "These environments consist of techniques as well as technologies, symbols as well as tools, information systems as well as machines."[32]

Such setting demonstrates its quantitative and qualitative properties, providing conditions for subsequent processes and changes. The ecological approach allows for appropriate location of each user in an integrated environment. In such integrated approach, both material and nonmaterial aspects can become indistinguishable and, as a result, the media should be perceived as material-nonmaterial, technology-content based and technical-social environment. Quoting Mark Deuze:

"This is not a life simply lived with more media than before the age of internet and mobile telephony. It is a way of living that fuses life with material and mediated conditions of living in ways that bypass the real or perceived dichotomy between such constituent elements of human existence."[33]

Such strong integration of the technological and content dimension which, according to Luciano Floridi,[34] takes place as a result of the re-ontologization of the infosphere caused by the development of ICT, enforces an integrated view which combines the material and the symbolic dimensions. This is in line with the school of media ecology investigating "the interactions of communications media, technology, technique, and processes with human feeling, thought, value, and behavior"[35] and assuming—similarly to the metathesis of mediatization—that "communication (. . .) is about mutation, and that the process of representation, signification, symbolization, and yes, mediation is in fact a process of transformation. (. . .) the study of communication is the study of change, as opposed to permanence."[36]

Setting up research on media saturation in media ecology does not mean adopting—what media ecologists are often accused of—determinism. First of all, as N. O. Finnemann emphasizes, "media are not agencies with separate intentionality."[37] R. Silverstone explains: "Technologies, it must be said, are enabling (and disabling) rather that determining. They emerge, exist and expire in a world not entirely of their own making."[38] Secondly, as M. Hansen notes, even M. McLuhan, a staunch defender of the inseparability of technology and culture, proved that technological determinism does not take place, because technology does not determine a situation. It cannot have such an impact since it is not positioned outside of culture. Similarly, continues M. Hansen, culture as such does not exist without technology, hence it cannot construct experiences on its own.[39] Hard determinism implies the passivity of an individual and his or her submission to influences, which entirely denies the bilateralism and the agility of the relationship between the media and the culture and society that can be observed. Thirdly, as M. Deuze rightly points out, media-centrism and technological determinism lead us to the illusion that there is a possibility of complete deactivation of the media or complete control over it.[40] Generally, one should agree with this statement. The degree of popularization and technological advancement excludes such a possibility on a global scale and to the full extent. However, it should be noted that in practice it is not intended to completely shut down or fully control the media, but rather to isolate from them in the material or symbolic dimension; in other words to separate certain aspects of life from mediated processes. The media, however, remain, act, saturate, and mediatize the reality. An individual can decide on the range of technologies he or she uses, the media practices implemented, and the degree of media presence in many spheres of his or her life. Although in many aspects, individuals have very restricted possibilities of limiting their own exposure to the media and not involving them in everyday life, numerous areas that are subject to increasingly frequent desaturation emerge. In line with the perspective of ecology (including media ecology), the environment is not only an environment that intervenes and makes "impact" but an area of human influence.

> "Organisms not only modify themselves to meet the demands of a changing environment, they also transform their environment to make it more favorable to their own survival and prosperity. (. . .) The media ecology approach to communication focuses on the means and methods, the techniques and technologies that bring about change. It therefore is concerned with the pragmatics of change, in addition to the substance of transformation."[41]

Reaching for the tradition of media ecology and in order to capture the mechanisms of mediatization, the research requires entering deeper into the nature and specificity of the media environment—or rather the relation of media elements with the user; looking at them from the micro and even the "nano" level—making a very close approach to individual elements of the technology and the phases of the processes completed by the user. The micro level can be broadly understood as activity of an individual using media technology (e.g., using a measuring technology during sport activity); whereas the 'nano' level includes concrete activities of an individual (e.g., manipulating with the device during a particular exercise to obtain particular results—be that sport effect or media effects). The analysis of the lowest levels helps explain mediated micro-management of activity.

However, limiting the analysis to the properties of the medium, including both content and technological, is insufficient. The key question is, which properties on the side of the medium, and which on the side of the active user, condition the specific mechanisms of mediatization; how these mechanisms work, ultimately leading to the mediatization of a specific domain of the individual and social world. Thus, it focuses on "the manner in which relations are set in motion through the communicative articulation of such mediatized worlds as a whole,"[42] but also through particular ways of using particular technologies.

In summary, the aim of research on mediatization is to identify the mechanisms of change (which may have its sources both inside and outside of the media) and their implications. For that purpose, media saturation is deployed as a necessary conceptual and methodological tool that allows to capture, record, and analyze those mechanisms.

Mediatization and Media Saturation

Research on the mechanisms of mediatization is part of "a new map of media research."[43] It is based on the resignation from centralization, through which N. Couldry understands the tendency in media studies (including research on production, distribution, and consumption) to focus on the largest media institutions.[44] As a result, other media areas are marginalized. Meanwhile, according to David Morley, nonmedia-centric media studies focus on the analysis of the interlacement of media processes and everyday life.[45]

> "It *can no longer* [emphasis in original] be a discipline that focuses only on the produced media of newspaper, TV, radio and film; it needs to deal with the diversity of contemporary media-mediated forms of communication. (. . .) In media cultures, saturated as they are with technical media oriented to reciprocity in communication, the classical mass media lose their pre-eminence (. . .)."[46]

Numerous studies on mediatization prove that this theory allows to abandon the perspective of a media center and, instead, to focus on the "media manifold"[47] and on the bi-directional relations between the media and various domains of individual and social worlds, in particular, focusing on users' everyday life. The relationship between a media change and a change in everyday life simply is "a core topic of mediatization."[48] So how should mediatization be treated and defined? N. Couldry proposes:

> "In general sociology, the term 'mediation' is used for any process of intermediation (such as money or transport). My concern here is however with the

term's specific uses in media research. Within media research, the term 'media-tion' can be used to refer simply to the act of transmitting something through the media, but here I have in mind a more substantive definition of the term which has received more attention in media research since the early 1990s. One crude definition of 'mediation'—in this substantive sense–is: the overall effect of media institutions existing in contemporary societies, the overall difference media make by being there in our social world."[49]

Without going into numerous terminology disputes about the distinction between terms such as mediation, mediatization, medialization, and even mediaization,[50] it should be stated that mediation is the kind of broker-age or agency in broadly understood communication, whereas mediatiza-tion—which takes place due to mediation combined with a transformation process—"implies that the maintenance and development of social life worlds, institutions and societies as well as the relationships between them, are becoming increasingly dependent on, and molded by media technologies, representations, and institutions."[51] The approach should not be limited to the meaning of media institutions and/or produced media content but should em-brace and concentrate on the specifics of media technology and mediated pro-cesses. Mediatization is actually the process of all intermediation. Through the mediation of the interaction with the device, during which information or raw data is exchanged, that information and data are subsequently used in universal human activity and social activities. Mediatization is the expression of "*second-order* [emphasis in original] complexity"[52] based on mediation, but also sufficient conditions of media environment, including its underlying quantitative and qualitative saturation.

Mediatization is a concept that enables the analysis of interrelations be-tween the changes in the media and communication as well as in culture and society,[53] and these relations are predominantly bilateral. The theory of mediatization distinguishes the institutional, social constructivist, and techno-logical approach[54] and its research perspectives are divided into institutional, cultural, material, and agency-oriented.[55]

Göran Bolin describes particular approaches.[56] The institutional approach is characterized by concentration on the media (mass media, especially news media) as institutions and their impact on other social institutions. Causality explanation, short historical perspective, and analyses concern mainly mezo level are typical for institutional approach.

According to G. Bolin, the social constructivist approach focuses on the study of the importance of the whole media environment. It combines the institutional and technological perspective. Here the media are part of the material and symbolic world, they are immersed in human practice.

"[I]nterplay between media, individual agency and the formation of structural consraints"[57] are studied. The analyses are dynamic, less causal, and concern mainly the mezo level.

The third technological approach derives from anthropology, linguistics, semantics, and the medium theory. It treats the media as technologies and codes. Researchers are interested in how technology structures the message. It is dominated by causality explanation.[58]

The main representative of the institutional approach is Stig Hjarvard, who points to the existence of the so-called modus operandi of the media[59] and refers to the so-called media logic.[60] "The term 'media logic' refers to the institutional and technological modus operandi of the media, including the ways in which media distribute material and symbolic resources and operate with the help of formal and informal rules."[61] The media intervene through their form, content, and organization.[62] They mediate indirectly (poorly) or directly (strongly). In the first case, they transform the existing activity, in the second case they transform the nonmediated element into mediated one, creating a kind of new activity, which has not existed before.[63]

The main representatives of the cultural, social, and constructivist approach are Fredrich Krotz, Andreas Hepp, and Nick Couldry. According to the first of them, mediatization is also treated as a "metaprocess that consists of a changing everyday life, of changing identity constructions and social relations, of a changing economy, democracy and leisure, of a changing culture and society as a whole."[64] Apart from individualization, commercialization, and globalization, mediatization is the fourth main metaprocess shaping modernity.[65] Andres Hepp with his concepts of molding forces[66] and communicative figurations[67] penetrates deeper into the mechanisms of change, wondering how they also occur at the mezo level. In his approach, he emphasizes the importance of contextualization of research.[68] The main question is what features of the media influence the given areas and what other changes co-exist with mediatization, and what makes media so important in human life. Nick Couldry, on the other hand, emphasizes the importance of two-way relations: media change the environment by transmitting "textual units" and the environment changes the conditions under which media function.[69] The cooperation between Andreas Hepp and Nick Couldry has resulted in the development of a phenomenological materialistic approach to mediatization, which is the basis for the analyses presented in this volume.

The technological approach includes the works of Jean Baudrillard, who develops mainly the concept of simulations of communication;[70] Marshall McLuhan and the whole ecological school: e.g., Neil Postman, Lance Strate, including the authors of medium theory, e.g., Joshua Meyrowitz. These researchers treat the media as multi-dimensional environments. They perceive changes and transformations in the long and medium term. Their considerations often become a part of critical media studies.

The saturation concept formulated in this study draws the most from the constructivist approach developed mainly by A. Hepp and F. Krotz and in the later period deepened in the phenomenological-material approach by A. Hepp and N. Couldry. In addition, especially in the empirical dimension, the study focuses on the technological approach. This is close to the directions of development of the theory of "mediatization as socio-technological transformations in the digital age,"[71] indicated by Sonia Livingstone and Peter Lunt. Focusing on the micro level, it also draws inspiration from the agency-oriented perspective:

"examining the microdynamics of mediatization processes (. . .). Such an actor- and agency-oriented approach puts actors' adaptation, innovation, collaborations, interactions, contradictions and resistance to media pressures and media technologies at the center of analysis. Paying attention to the micro- and specifics of interactions, relations, structures, motives, and activities related to the media, provides possibilities to analyze more closely the ways in which individual as well as collective actors act when they conform to and/or confront mediatization's behavioral scripts."[72]

Mediatization is the "process of increasing deepening of technology-based interdependence."[73] Technological interdependencies do not only pertain to the collective, social dimension, but also to the specific daily endeavors of every individual. As previously stated, research on mediatization cannot be limited only to what is collective and collectively constructed, but it also should find room for individual perspective: for personal motivations, goals, and effects of actions, which should make them closer to technological and agency-oriented approaches. In addition to social worlds, the private worlds of individual users' lives or aspects of their mediated activity that remain the domain of private life should be examined. Clearly, both the individual and social perspectives overlap and are naturally intertwined. However, one must remember that not all mediated activities are simultaneously socially communicated; they often remain at the level of interaction with the device or at the level of the user's communication with himself or herself. Therefore, it seems reasonable to highlight how "a society in media is at once individual and interconnected as it is both embodied and virtual."[74] The theory of mediatization provides the basics for that as it is open to continuous change and modification; it is multi-threaded and exhibits internal diversity. It also includes the advanced variant, the so-called "deep mediatization," which pertains not only to how media shapes the basic elements of the social world, but also how they are connected at all levels.[75] Shaping up, defining the smallest elements of social and individual worlds is mediated through technology. The goal of this study is to obtain insight into the properties of these individual elements and relations between them. Deep mediatization does not just mean that "the very elements and building blocks from which *sense* (emphasis in original) of the social is constructed become themselves based on technologically based processes of mediation;"[76] but highlights the fact that the saturating media technologies shape the mechanics of everyday practices: the ways and methods of their implementation. Therefore, the integration of elements of the constructivist, technical and agency-oriented approach is necessary.

Regardless of the perspective adopted,[77] the aspects observed at particular levels of mediatization require further specification with the focus on the possibilities of viewing and analyzing these change mechanisms, including micro-mechanisms. This stems from the fact that the phenomena occurring at the social mezzo and macro level are possible due to the micro level phenomena; similarly, transformations at the individual levels co-depend on those levels, too. The particularity of mediated individual activities determines social behaviors, protocols and actions. A reverse relationship, when the nature of mediatized social phenomena determines the course of particular human activities, can also be observed.

THE CONCEPT OF MEDIA SATURATION

Media researchers emphasize the importance of media omnipresence and their integration with everyday life.[78] It seems to be obvious, both for users and researchers. However, much less importance, if any, is attached to the volume of this presence and the mechanisms of media integration with life. Also, specifying the areas of media presence in life is not enough to assess its saturation levels. It appears that there is a need to determine the distribution of this presence, its degree, the scope of mediated activities, and lastly, the qualitative specificity of the mechanisms that enable and reinforce the possible ubiquity of the media.

A common approach to quantitative measurement of the volume of media presence relies on calculating time spent with the media, which has been adapted since the beginning of mass media domination.[79] It is an attempt to assess the saturation of the actual people's life with media, but only in the dimension of time. Such studies show how media seize the modern man's time. However, they offer very little insights into the mechanisms of media penetration of physical space. They rarely take into account the material and processual dimension affecting the process of the environment and human activity saturation.

The strive to capture saturation of the environment and human action methodically and with the use of both quantitative and qualitative methods, requires the introduction of new terms in order to "explain some phenomenon that previously escaped explanation."[80] It also requires a new research method that can be applied universally and used for comparative research, including research that enables to grasp changes over time.

Abductive Reasoning: From Meta-theory to Subject Theory and Vice Versa

The method used to determine media saturation in more detail from the perspective of mediatization is abduction.[81] Abduction reasoning indicates possible conditions that explain the relationship between the rule and the result.[82] Its form is presented in the following way:

> We observe the surprising phenomenon of C.
> If A were true, then the existence of C would be obvious.
> Hence there's a reason to suspect that A is true.[83]

In abductive reasoning "we try to connect phenomena (seemingly) distant from each other"[84]—what is claimed is not directly observed, but mediated by other processes of reasoning, which allows us to accumulate experiences, thanks to which we make new discoveries.[85]

According to L. Schofield Clark, it is actually research on mediatization that requires the above reasoning, which utilizes induction, deduction and "creative element that looks to unifying conceptions (. . .). Analogical reasoning involves presenting an argument by drawing comparisons between a new concept and something already understood and thus can identify concepts so as to pint toward the future."[86] The quintessence of this type of reasoning is a thought experiment, followed by a methodological and empirical test. Abduction serves as the initial stage of investigation after which predictions are created by facilitates modeling of explanatory procedures.[87]

The concept of media saturation, integrating the existing findings of studies on mediatization, in particular within meta-theoretical context, is a proposal requiring methodological and empirical testing of a specific everyday life area. Resulting from observations of both progressing mediatization as well as the symptoms of following demediatization, it is assumed that the particular degree and nature of saturation of the environment and human activity characterizes mediatization, i.e., in cases of deficient quantitative saturation and insufficient parameters of qualitative saturation, mediatization does not occur. Similarly, given high degrees of saturation and particular characteristics of saturation, demediatization does appear. Hence, and in line with the formula of Charles Pierce, there are grounds for suspecting that the volume and nature of media saturation are crucial for mediatization to take place. From a methodological perspective this means that saturation is a property, or rather a parameter, characterizing mediatization.

Theorizing Media Saturation

Applying the abduction procedure followed by methodological and empirical testing of the media saturation corresponds with the postulates advocated by the mediatization researchers, including, but not limited to, the need "to get different 'grounded theories' of how media communicative change and sociocultural change are interlaced with each other,"[88] and developing a general theory of mediatization on the basis of them.

According to the typology formed by F. Krotz and explained by A. Hepp, there are three main types of theory: mathematical; substantive; and metatheories.[89] The first category refers to "a delimited domain of mathematically formurable (functional) relationships"[90] and is based on quantitative methods. The second "typify a delimited domain of phenomena in terms of structure and process and is based on qualitative methods"[91] while substantive theories "develop theory-laden categorical systems through the comparative analysis of relevant material."[92] Finally, metatheories are described as: "narratives that go beyond particular domains of phenomena and which tend to general explanation,"[93] built of substantive and mathematical theories.

Mediatization is a kind of metatheory. In order to pose the problem of quantitative and qualitative specifics of mediatization mechanisms at various levels (from micro through mezzo to macro levels)—and thus to further clarify the problem of media saturation—it is necessary to properly locate it within the metatheory of mediatization to enable the empirical exploration of the phenomenon. Following that, it is imperative to adhere to the methodological framework of empirical research on the cultures of mediatization, beginning with the development of theory, through decentralization and patterns analysis, concluding in transcultural comparison.[94]

According to A. Hepp, theoretical framework should be developed as a result of generating theory, and not as a result of testing it, which is consistent with the assumptions of, for example, grounded theory. Barney Glaser and Anselm Strauss distinguished substantive and formal theories[95] with the latter seen as a prompt for the development of metatheories in the perspective of F. Krotz, who stated that formal theory "derived from the comparative analysis of key categories identified from among a range of substantive theories."[96] Therefore, the groundwork for the development of metatheories is based on the effectiveness of connections between substantive theories.[97] In the presented study, the concept of media saturation will be separated and then defined with the help of the abduction method while drawing from the achievements of media studies, especially research focusing on mediatization.

It will be grounded in the hitherto research findings and related to the needs and challenges faced by contemporary media research.

Next, the study methodology will be determined. Based on empirical research, an attempt will be made to identify patterns of mediation and mediatization. Their subsequent analysis will focus on the identification of typical forms in a particular cultural context based on the research of diverse individual phenomena.[98] The emergence of typical forms and their concentration is necessary for the occurrence of a specific cultural pattern to emerge. This can be achieved by media saturation analysis, allowing for the separation of repetitive, to some extent constituted, media saturation patterns of individual fields, areas, and objects; and schemes of media saturation processes, including patterns of interaction and co-interaction of the media, which take place through media saturation and lead to mediatization. The last element of the study will refer to comparative studies[99] to draw parallels between various media-sports worlds.

Most importantly, therefore, there is a need for theoretical and methodological arrangement of current literature and findings on media saturation, in order to define media saturation correctly and to examine it interdependently. The next necessary step is to determine the methods examining the quantitative and qualitative aspects of the process in a methodical manner, and the tests, thus providing the potential basis for the comparison of the subsequent results.

Media Study-related Origins of Media Saturation

It seems appropriate to begin with the analysis of the context in which the term "media saturation" occurs in current studies; its significance and the potential of its application in research on mediatization. Like many other concepts used in media studies, the genesis of the term is strongly interdisciplinary. The concept of saturation is used, for example, in chemistry (saturation of one substance with the other, e.g., water with salt, liquid with gas),[100] medicine (blood saturation with oxygen),[101] art (intensity of color),[102] and marketing (using available means to win the market).[103] In technical and natural sciences, saturation stands either for the act itself: the state of being saturated, or the conversion of an unsaturated compound into a saturated one; or depicts the state of maximum impregnation.[104] Depending on the discipline or a specific phenomenon, saturation can be identified as or distinguished from satiation, i.e., reaching the state of maximum dissolution, absorption, accommodation, or storing of one element in another.[105]

In media studies, media saturation appears very often as a descriptive, not an analytical, concept. It is freely used and interpreted without restrictions, which does not ease analysis or interpretation, but can lead to methodological confusion. There is a diverse array of definitions, as well as the freedom to apply them without offering a comprehensive explanation.

The problem of definitional freedom was criticized by Jay Newell. As he rightly pointed out "the term *media saturation* [emphasis in original] is an occasionally used but undefined assumption of social critics."[106] The author refers to researchers publishing their key papers in the 1980s, defining them as postmodern, e.g., Angela McRobbie, Jean Baudrillard or Todd Gitlin.[107] Although these authors do not define media saturation precisely, J. Newell synthesizes their standpoints using such terms as: "insertion of mass media into private, formerly unmediated spaces,"[108] "expansion of mass media as the mechanism by which global companies would overwhelm and redirect individual thought,"[109] "supersaturation (. . .) media exposure that was continuous and overwhelming."[110] Current critical thought on saturation—although only present in indirect studies—includes research focused on broadly understood overload, in the information, visual, and technological dimensions. Todd Gitlin, Neil Postman, Paul Virillo, and Kenneth Gergen[111] are specified as "subscribers to the 'saturation' thesis."[112]

J. Newell separates the critical thought from the results of empirical studies on saturation, which, however, in their definition assumptions, appear to be equally divergent and not always clear. This list includes Faust Izcaray's proposal from 1980, defining media saturation as a function of media availability in particular regions. Based on his research, the author identified areas with high, medium, and low media saturation, which he translated into knowing public affairs.[113] Following this path, John Sherry developed a definition of a media-saturated country, which "is typified by a large number of competing media, a large number of channels within those media, and a large variety of messages on those channels."[114] According to J. Newell, mass media research focuses only on their accessibility, not on effects, and in cases where it does reach beyond accessibility, studies focus predominantly on consumption.[115] Despite the indirectly formulated postulate to broaden the perspective, the author himself also adopts limited optics in his research and the conclusions from his study mainly pertain to the usage of electronic media[116] and "the apparent paradox of media consumption change."[117] What is more important, however, is that all of the mentioned research projects, including J. Newell's proposal, are focused merely on researching the perception of media content, but not the use of media technology, its physical presence, material specificity, and diverse applications, which generate particular individual and social effects. A similar situation can be observed in research on the consumers' exposure to the media. Todd Gitlin rightly shows that most of this type of studies pertains to the time spent on watching or listening to media and the issue of being exposed to the media remains debatable due to a variety of factors, including "rapt attention, vague awareness, oblivious coexistence, and all possible shadings in between."[118]

The concept of media saturation can also be found in the work of media experts investigating socio-cultural impact of the media from a broad perspective.[119] Neither the authors of textbooks synthesizing media science shy away from applying this concept.[120] Typically, researchers who use the term of media saturation—without its wider explanation—often juxtapose it with the concept of mediatization or position it within the context of mediatization. That could indicate either their awareness of the relationships between the two phenomena, or a particular research intuition of mediatization and media saturation being closely intertwined. Less than a decade ago, N. Couldry signaled the problem of "media saturation," seen as a peculiar degree of media presence in the environment. He postulated then to resign from using the term "media saturation," stating that it allows to "capture *media density* [emphasis in original] in selected contemporary social environments, but does not cover the multi-dimensional character of the transformation of society through media."[121]

The advanced works in the field of mediatization use that concept particularly frequently. It seems that the reflections on media studies published hitherto lack a proper, precise definition of saturation and a proposal that would integrate the structural and processual dimensions; quantitative and qualitative; individual and social; and finally, material and nonmaterial. There is also a need to expand the scope of research on mediatization,[122] mainly constituting of research on the content, by shifting its focus to the remaining dimensions of the media and their more precise parameterization, i.e., expression and explanation in the form of quantitative and qualitative parameters.

In papers coming from other strands of media studies, such as studies on political communication, a clear definition of media saturation is also often missing. Tim O'Sullivan, Bryan Dutton, and Philip Rayner distinguish two ways of capturing the media saturation: as a measurement of "amounts of time that we spend in media-related activities, largely forms and practices of media consumption" and examination of "available evidence which charts either the diffusion or penetration of media hardware or the circulation of particular media products."[123] Author Bogustawa Ostrowska's definition was formulated for the purpose of research on political and public communication, but it appears to be relatively universal and open to development in the course of further research into the phenomenon also in other areas of communication and everyday life: "media saturation of society is a process which progresses along with the development of communication technology and easy access to it, consists in "saturating" the society with an increasing number of technical media means and intertwining it with a very dense message network, which in turn causes addiction of citizens to information media."[124] The quoted definition is of a critical nature as it indicates a negative effect of the phenomenon (since its addictive nature is mentioned), but what is more important is that not only the content but also the technological dimension of the media and its significance for saturation are highlighted. The author emphasizes not only the importance of content, but also of material communication tools, as did Tim O'Sullivan, Bryan Dutton, and Philip Rayner.[125]

"The dynamic development of new communication and information technologies systematically enriches the forms of political communication. (. . .) Intensification of contacts and the bilateral flow of information from political broadcasters to citizens and the reverse, contributes to the development of democracy. In the countries with the highest degree of media saturation and when state-of-the-art transmission techniques are used, there are discussions on communication democracy as on a higher form of development."[126]

Although that reflection concerns only the political importance of saturation, its individual effect is still noticed. Similarly, although the stress falls mainly on informational messages, which is understandable since the mediatization of politics is described, the general term "message network" permits expanding the field of reflection on other types of mediatizing content. It also turns out to be the key to the statement of T. O'Sullivan, B. Dutton, and P. Rayner that "we inhabit cultures and worlds which have been described as *media saturated* [emphasis in original]."[127]

On this occasion, it should be noted that the descriptive nature and interpretational liberty are not something unique in the case of this particular concept. Similar discrepancies and discretion apply to other commonly used concepts in media studies and they are not exclusively typical for media researchers, but also for representatives of other disciplines. For example, in cultural studies,[128] linguistics,[129] or pedagogy,[130] the concept of media saturation is also cited without in-depth analysis, although far-reaching and mainly critical conclusions are drawn based on the notion that media saturation occurs.[131]

SATURATION AS A MEDIATIZATION PARAMETER

The perspective of media saturation presented in hitherto studies only scarcely fit into the problem of media technologies saturation of the environment and human activity. In most cases, they are either theoretical-critical, or empirically limited by a narrow research perspective, focusing mainly on media content. There is a need for a more broadly grounded approach that allows empirical studies of various spheres of human life. Referring to previous studies focused on the theory of mediatization potential, the concept of media saturation should respond to the basic assumptions of this theory and the challenges it is currently faced with. N. Couldry and A. Hepp postulate that new analytical tools, allowing for research of the distinctive characteristics of the relatively newly formed digital media environment and its relationship with media users, should be developed.[132] The development of media saturation studies also responds to the postulate of N. O. Finnemann pertaining to the need to integrate new parameters with the concept of the media, and subsequently to contribute to the development of the mediatization theory.[133] Media saturation, therefore, acts both as a conceptual tool and a methodological approach, providing concrete indications for empirical research. Research occurs through "analytic view that tends to dismantle mediatization into other processes."[134]

In line with Knut Lundby's viewpoint that mediatization is characterized by different modes of mediatization, which are comprised of "parameters within which the transformations could be analyzed,"[135] media saturation appears to be one of the key factors contributing to the study change. K. Lundby assumes that those parameters "may derive from characteristics of the media environment, point to mechanisms of change (. . .). They may also depend on technological affordances, as with digitization."[136]

While identifying saturation as a parameter of mediatization, it can be defined as a quantitatively and qualitatively assessed presence and the functioning of the entire media infrastructure, devices, and their content within human environment, which comprise of a large part of people's activities and thus form the basis of mediatization.[137]

Taking into account the aforementioned dual nature of technology[138] (artifactual and technology in action), two aspects of media saturation should be distinguished: structural and processual.[139] Structural media saturation (in other words, technological saturation) corresponds to the artifactual dimension of media technology. Its structural dimension results from interpreting the structure as resources and principles that are applicable both in social[140] and individual practice. It corresponds with the saturation of a given object, area, space, and consequently, social worlds and diversified domains of people's everyday life.[141] While infrastructural and technical aspects of media can condition as well as transform the environment, object, area, and space, and, as a result, the social worlds and domains of human life, it simultaneously succumbs to their influences too.

Processual media saturation corresponds to the technology-in-practice dimension—particular, significant applications of technologies that determine the transformation of everyday life. It is the saturation of people's activities by technologically mediated processes. Quantitatively and qualitatively suitable conditions of processual saturation enable the "transformation process," consisting of "communication change the social and cultural environments (. . .) as well as the relationships that participants, both individual and institutional, have to that environment and to each other."[142] If exposed to a particular spectrum, degree, and quality of saturation, resulting in sufficient saturation with media technology and mediated processes, both in terms of quantity and quality, mutual and significant transformation may occur.

It is important, therefore, to determine the most beneficial approach to the analysis of media saturation seen as a parameter of mediatization in the new technologies development era and its quantitative and qualitative measurement. Some of the findings within the theory of mediatization emphasize media content and its social effects by accentuating the importance of media content for generating a particular meaning by individuals and its objectivization[143] and social reification.[144] A. Hepp, while defining media cultures, ventures beyond the content to some extent by drawing attention to the fact that "primary meaning[145] resources are mediated through technical communications media, which are 'molded' by these processes in specifically different ways."[146] The form—and often the content of media messages—results from the structure of technology, its functionalities, design, affordances. Therefore, focusing exclusively or mainly on the content does not provide an answer to the question of how proper media saturation results in mediatization. It is in the material properties of technology and the specifics of mediated processes that the mechanisms of mediatization are found. The content is complementary, and sometimes only accompanying; due to the technological possibilities available to users it can be generated, transmitted, archived, and analyzed by them. Thus, the media saturation study mainly pertains to the volume and nature of the presence of technology in everyday life and its implications.

Mediatization Mechanisms

It can be said that studies on media saturation focus on the mechanics of mediatization and are intended to reveal the ways of operation of mediatization mechanisms, which include relationships between the infrastructure and devices, the content, and ways of use. Media saturation may constitute one of the concepts, which will reinforce the theory of mediatization enabling "to 'pick out' purported key mechanisms and forces within a complex whole."[147]

Particular mechanisms that intensify, repeat, continually expand their scope, and thus mediatize a given sphere of everyday life, can be observed in media practice. In order for these mechanisms to reveal themselves, specific elements in the build of a technology and appropriate connections between these mechanisms and content are required. When activated and combined with the repetition of their action, they generate change and thus technology becomes a kind of a media vehicle. In this context, K. Lundby recalls the concept of Pitirim Sorokin's "material vehicles" of change, which can be either physical or symbolic, or physical and symbolic at the same time.[148] This observation largely corresponds with the nature of media technologies, which, in their basic dimension, are essentially material tools. It is worth noting that, at times, their symbolic function is emphasized, particularly due to their unique capabilities, or when the mediation in transmitting the content.

While P. Sorokin writes, "physical conductors work in gestures and body movements, in sound waves, light and color, in thermal and mechanical forms of energy,"[149] "'electrical and radio conductors,"[150] K. Lundby adds that vehicles might be also digital. "*Physical* [emphasis in original] conductors are those in which the physical qualities of the vehicle are used to modify the state of mind and the overt actions of another."[151] Sound, light, and color, pantomime (nonverbal, body language-based), thermal, mechanical, chemical, electrical, and radio waves can also act as vehicles.[152] On the other hand, "*symbolic* [emphasis in original] conductors exert an influence not so much by virtue of their physical properties as by virtue of the symbolic meaning attached to them."[153]

According to K. Lundby, media vehicles facilitate interaction.[154] They act as managers, conductors in externalization, objectivization, and socialization of meanings, whereas mediatization takes place, "when various media impact people's life horizons and form a basis for a significant part of the social interaction within a certain domain, thus becoming a 'mediatized world.'"[155]

"We need to understand mediatization and interaction in the span between agency and structure, between acts and the format or setting they relate to."[156] It should be added that mediatization occurs due to vehicles of media technologies, which not only enable social interaction but above all an interaction with the entire system provided by the device and, in consequence, an interaction with resources, especially those generated by the users themselves: data, content; mediated thoughts; and actions. Media technologies are vehicles of social and individual change; mediators of life worlds and tools for mediatizing social worlds. They are of a particular dual nature: physical and symbolic; they act as operational tools and containers, transmitters, and content creators at the same time. And due to these inter-relations, they facilitate mediatization.

These peculiar mechanics have a binary character: both structural and simultaneously processual, including discursive processes[157]—where communication is only one of the mediated processes.

Studies on media saturation require penetration into their nature. On the one hand, it is necessary to reveal the internal mechanisms (relations between structures and internal processes) of the media, which determine the operation, functionalities, effectiveness of the media, etc. in order to understand the way they work. On the other hand, it is necessary to examine the external mechanisms of the media, that is, the forces formed between the media structure and various activities of everyday life. Research on the mechanics of mediatization strives, therefore, to answer the question of how media saturation in the quantitative and qualitative sense co-determines the wider sociocultural changes and how these changes decide about the media change. The role of context is very significant here as media saturation allows to explain mediatization via the analysis of the qualitative and quantitative implication of the internal media mechanisms and their elements in the contextualized activities undertaken users.

As A. Hepp states, media "do reveal in their entirety a *particular potential for action*; this we can call the *moulding forces* [emphasis in original] of media (. . .)."[158] It should be pointed out, however, that the potential for action can be realized due to the appropriate (in the quantitative and qualitative sense) media saturation. This potential lies in structures (their shape, properties) and generated processes (their dynamics, their course) and relations between them (e.g., in the form of affordances, which lead from appropriate structures through processes to actions, resulting in specific outcomes).

Every aspect of social world, area of activity, and sphere of life is characterized by a distinct peculiarity. For each area, it is required to determine a way in which molding can be investigated.[159] The aim of the media saturation concept is to enrich the ability of broadening knowledge about internal and external conditioning of the shaping forces. Media saturation serves as an analytical and conceptual foundation for that.

Quantitative and Qualitative Studies on Media Saturation

"Can, then, mediatization at all be described as a quantitative growth of media influence, or is it rather a set of qualitative shifts in how media relate to other spheres (. . .)?"[160] Mediatization has distinctive quantitative and qualitative aspects. Both aspects must be tested simultaneously in order to get a full view of the transformation of a given sphere. Research on media saturation as the parameter of mediatization provides an opportunity to approach specific values and characteristics of phenomena and their processes.

It allows to define them in a quantitative and qualitative sense. A condition for successful application of the concept in research practice lies in the exact specification of the parameter.

It is possible to examine quantitative and qualitative aspects of both structural and processual saturation. In the first case, analysis determines the spectrum and degree of saturation of the environment with technologies, focusing on a specific area, object, social world, everyday life domain (quantitative aspect) and exploring the features of technologies such as infrastructure capabilities, functionalities, design, and affordances of a device (qualitative aspect). Similarly, it is possible to determine the quantitative and qualitative aspects of processual saturation. It encompasses a spectrum of processes, and thus the sequence of activities based on mediated activities, and the degree of saturation with these processes is calculated. Determining the quality of mediated processes is possible through studying processes' features and the mechanisms that they shape, which condition mediatization.

A spectrum should be understood as the scope of technologies applied and mediated processes implemented. We can distinguish the ideal spectrum (all existing technologies, all possible mediated processes) and the real spectrum (hereinafter referred to as the spectrum), which is, defined on the basis of preliminary research, the range of actually used technologies in a particular activity and the mediated processes realized within that activity, which can be examined in a given time and place.

The saturation degree should be understood as the quantified value corresponding to the use of the available spectrum of technologies and processes potential. The saturation level may take many different shapes depending on the problem and the purpose of research.[161] The adopted research perspective, the problems, and objectives of the research, will determine other aspects for measurement and description. Each time, the problems of spectrum and saturation degree will require operationalization to serve the needs of a given research program. In terms of qualitative aspects of saturation, the issue of characterizing the specificity of saturation will be even more sophisticated and require contextualization.

Examining media saturation can consist of a three-fold determination of changes in saturation with the media, i.e., changes in a given time period, space, or range, analogously to the examination of the aspects of mediatization according to F. Krotz.[162] However, within mediatization analysis, individual comparisons pertain to:

- changes in the number of technologically mediatized forms of communication;
- changes in their location; and

- changes in the number of relationships and social institutions that are subject to technological mediatization.

While investigating media saturation, changes are examined within the following scope:

- saturation range (the spectrum of technologies and mediated processes in a given activity);
- saturation degree (measured, for example, by the scale to which particular tools are used, the occurrence of particular processes);
- the specificity of cultural, psychological, and social processes and phenomena that occur or are transformed due to media saturation, but also co-determine the media change.

Within the first aforementioned perspective on changes, the range of technologies available to people is an "aggregate of accessible communications media (. . .) the totality of communications media available at one point in space-time."[163] From the pool of constantly growing number of available technologies, a user creates an individual constellation of platforms that are engaged in particular daily activities. Secondly, the selection of particular technologies, and their number determines the degree of technological saturation of the individual or collective practice. It allows to determine what technologies dominate in the "media manifold"[164] in terms of frequency of use, diversity of use, their meaning in practice, etc. Lastly, the quantitative evaluation serves as a starting point to evaluate the rationale behind certain media technologies importance and their application in practice.

Qualitative saturation examination involves studying the relationship between structures, messages, and processes. It allows to answer the question of how technological saturation (with a given spectrum and achieving a certain degree of saturation) and processual saturation (including discursive saturation) mediatize a given sphere of life. Hence, qualitative examination of media saturation includes three main elements and relationships between them: technology, content (form and substance), and user's activity.

The Problem of Media Desaturation

The ever-increasing presence of new media technologies in numerous aspects of human life, resulting in subordinating many aspects of everyday activity to the media technologies, can trigger users' strive to protect and isolate some aspects of life from mediation, and at times from far-reaching mediatization. Users claim 'the right to disconnect.'"[165] The constant presence of new, handheld, multifunctional, converged media in the human environment causes diverse cultural and social implications while also activating resistance to changes and, every so often, a drive to minimize their impact or to reverse them. N. Couldry and A. Hepp assume that, in principle, demediatization is impossible. By definition, media constitutes a reference framework for all activities, including those that are not mediatized. To some extent this view is supported by M. Deuze, claiming that we live in the media, and not with the media,[166] and we are actually dealing with the "supersaturation of media messages and machines in households, workplaces, shopping malls, bars and restaurants, an all the other in-between spaces of today's world."[167] This begs a question: is there no escape from the media? Is demediatization impossible?

It is not a folly to assume, somewhat paradoxically, that even if widespread and deep demediatization had taken place with a subsequent retreat from changes resulting from the mutual transformation of the media and other spheres of human life, this would indicate the power of mediatization. Its significance, its implications would potentially be so profound and significant to people that it would prompt them to restore the old order. In other words, users would take action in response to the presence and power of the media. Their lives would still be mediatized, however, as they would not reach the state from before the occurrence of mediatization changes; changes that leave irreversible psychological, social, and cultural, as well as economic and even environmental impact. It would be a new state, yet still burdened with experiences and implications of mediatization. Therefore, due to the power of its strength and proliferation, mediatization would continue: demonstrated in the ways of thinking, norms and principles, expectations and actions, though it is difficult to predict what exact shape such reality would take.

Undoubtedly, contemporary life outside the mediatized world is restricted to monks, hermits, indigenous tribes, and some individuals, families, and communities that decide to leave the technologized areas—and thus, to a large extent, the modern civilization—and live "in the wilderness."[168] It is possible to observe and experience individual, temporary periods of isolation, which, according to N. Couldry and A. Hepp, condemn thinking about escaping from mediatization to failure. The authors consider limiting their own media accessibility (e.g., by being in places that block a wireless signal, etc.) as meaningless search for "oases of de-mediatization,"[169] because they all lead "to a return, to a re-absorption into media which in turn acts to confirm the depth of mediatization 'after all.'[170] This thought is continued by A. Hepp together with Uwe Hasebrink, stating that avoidance of mediation is an expression of deep mediatization which includes:

"the practice of bringing one's attention to things occurring in the present moment, beyond any mediated communication—is less about any durable containment of mediatization: it is rather an expression that deep mediatization includes spaces of self-reflection and controlled escape in order to remain manageable for us as human beings."[171]

Such statements, especially in the context of particular phenomena observed in this study, give rise to a whole series of questions. If the vast majority of the civilized world's citizens do not decide on permanent media isolation, then does demediatization not (at some even marginal level) occur? Does temporary suspension of mediation indicate a particular human weakness? Are specific actions (and not just a reflection on the situation) an expression of mediatization or rather a practical reaction leading to isolation and withdrawal? Is the suspension of processes that are decisive for the possible demediatization a cry for long-term or permanent separation from specific processes, operations, and activities? Are demediatization attempts confined within gradual isolation of aspects of everyday life; but not aimed at leading to its totality? Is it because we cannot imagine the existence of even partially demediatized world? The examples cited by N. Couldry, A. Hepp, and U. Hasebrink do confirm that people have the need for demediatization, but they do not seem to be able to fully carry it out. Paradoxically, and potentially due to even deeper mediatization, the manner of fulfilling this need will become clearer.

Some researchers are aware of the changing nature of trends, both those "long-term evolutionary processes" and "sharp epochal shifts" and ponder the possibility of demediatization[172] or identify moments when some social institutions become "more dominated by other types of steering logic."[173] This, according to Johan Fornäs, arises from a nonlinear but sinusoidal course of mediatization. "Strong waves of mediatization induce quantitative and qualitative shifts on many different levels. In between, minor shifts sometimes strengthen the role of media and at other times challenge them or integrate into other sociocultural configurations."[174] If we assume that mediatization "indicates a cumulative *increase* [emphasis in original] in the embeddedness of society by communication media,"[175] then every attempt to decrease its growing influence or proliferation and consolidation in everyday practices is already a signal of potential demediatization. We should also take into consideration that a media change is both incremental and radical. Since "evolutions and revolutions will always shade one into the other,"[176] the dominance of one tendency is not mutually exclusive to a change in the opposite direction.

Demediatization, similar to mediatization, is of a discrete and complex nature. It results from the relationship between various areas of human life: social, cultural, economic, psychological, and environmental. It does not take the form of a revolution. It does not happen suddenly, and there is no rampant course of action as there are no conditions for that either. Demediatization is a residual and sluggish process and it is a response to the dominance and primacy of media technologies in most areas of human life. Currently, and to a large extent, it is part of the numerous takes on the logic or grammar of mediatization, if only because the ubiquity and diversity of media technologies forces the usage of new technologies, including those facilitating isolation.[177] Demediatization, perceived as a retreat, an attempt at restoring the unmediatized order in the selected areas of human life, and thus minimizing the power of mediatization (after all, there is no mediatization without mediation), is a step toward demediatization of certain spheres of life. It occurs as a result of the demediation and gradual reduction of the quantitative and qualitative presence of media technologies in human life, that is, by the way of media desaturation.

The problem of technological desaturation seems disputable, mainly due to the ubiquity of media technology and its apparent inescapability.[178] However, despite the inevitable and, as it seems, irreversible mediatization, it is "external to media life."[179] And although media desaturation is difficult to implement in practice, the media is not "unavoidable"[180] They can be reflected in the empirically observed process of technological and processual desaturation discussed further in this volume.[181] As far as "they are impossible to (completely) escape from, and cannot be (completely) switched off,"[182] media desaturation of objects, spaces, and domains of life is possible, which points to the defragmenting nature of the processes of mediatization, and potentially also its reversal.

Although mediatization results in the media sphere and other spheres of human life, mutual transformation, at the material level the possibility to separate and isolate the material media—and thus the demediation of selected processes—is possible. Currently, the separation is insufficient for the general social demediatization to emerge (after all, the question remains whether people want it), but it is powerful enough to demediate and detechnologize a particular sphere of a person's life; it can take place when an individual does not use media technology in a particular sphere of life, does not implement mediated processes and does not refer an activity to the media-shaped, socially-shared meaning of this activity and its components. Also, everyday life practices are at times not mediated. Concrete, everyday situations are transformed into unmediated alternatives or, rather, restored to their unmediated status. The everyday life of ordinary users is an exemplification of important tendencies that are present in culture and it is symptomatic of emerging new socio-cultural tendencies. Mediatization is a metaprocess from which a complete escape is impossible, but ordinary media users can take steps and actions to reverse the imposed order. Thus, research on demediatzation aims to "capture and recognize the active role of actors subjected to mediatization pressures. The active, skillful, and resourceful responses to mediatization pressures (. . .) to describe and understand the changes and dynamics of mediatization itself."[183] This involves the need to explain what demediation and desaturation is, and what results potential demediatization of human life could yield, seen as a profound retransformation, not as mere disappearing of the media.[184]

PHYSICAL ACTIVITY AS A SATURATED AND MEDIATIZED DOMAIN OF EVERYDAY LIFE

Mediatization cannot be examined "in total," but should focus on the specificity of a particular field or domain.[185] Due to the diversity of contexts, it has to be analyzed in relation to specific areas, spheres, precisely: "life-worlds."[186] F. Krotz and A. Hepp point out to paradigmatic traditional phenomenological and interactionist sources of the studies on worlds (media-worlds, life-worlds) and perceive everyday life-world as a natural, social, cultural, and "accepted without question"[187] world.

> "Media and the messages they broadcast can consequently be said to penetrate more deeply into everyday consciousness. And newer interactive or participatory media (e.g., mobile phones, texting, blogging, etc.) increasingly *inter*penetrate (emphasis in original) everyday activity. Media in this sense profoundly influence the realm of everyday, unstructured understandings and activities (or what German philosophers and sociologists have termed the *Lebenswelt* (emphasis in original) or lifeworld."[188]

The life-world of modern man is built out of smaller worlds, and it is characterized by the existence of a super-territorial communication network diversified in scale (from small, local, to large), interlaced and continuous segmentation, reconstruction and transgression from one world to another.[189] "People live in relations to a plurality of life-worlds (. . .); each of these spaces requires differing forms of communicative action, and as communication media have been developed to address these communicative practices, their protocols and their use give shape to the life-worlds we inhabit."[190] The multitude of everyday activities is subject to media saturation and mediatization. Domains are diverse, also in terms of the media to which they are exposed. The world of physical activity, exercise, and amateur sport (and its individual disciplines), is an example of the domain that forms everyday life, in which smaller worlds can be distinguished and "defined by a shared practical orientation of the human acting within this domain."[191] Those are cultural and socio-media worlds, which integrate within a specific domain of life individual and social media practices. Within them, we can distinguish micro-worlds, which by combining particular forms of activity and particular media technologies deployed in the practice of physical activity, lead to the formation of new patterns while engaging in a given sport discipline. They can be defined as mediatized worlds and sub-worlds. Following Anselm Strauss's concept of "social worlds."[192] A. Hepp proposed that mediatized worlds are "everyday manifestation of media culture."[193] Their size does not result from the scope, but from the complexity of elements corresponding to their focus. They can be comprised of large, complex worlds, as well as small, simple worlds and sub-worlds.[194]

The area of sport and physical activity shows high dynamics and strong integration with the media world.[195] Sport is a "hot spot," it defines "new dynamics for the future"[196] and, as a sphere susceptible to changes and in-novations, it dictates the direction of trends, tendencies, fashions, as well as changes in relations between media and other spheres of life.

Research into the mediatization of sport focuses primarily on professional sport. They are of interest to researchers because of their strong, synergistic economic relations ("media sport content economy"[197]) and socio-cultural relations, sometimes referred to as "sport-media nexus."[198] For a long time they were mainly limited to research into the relationship between sport and television.[199] Kirsten Frandsen is a key representative of the mediatization ap-proach in research into professional sport, whose work falls mainly within the institutional approach and concerns both sport broadcasting,[200] the organiza-tion of major sporting events (such as Tour de France[201]), and the mediatiza-tion of sports organizations,[202] recently also amateur sport and the importance of new technologies in it.[203]

Mediatization, however, impacts not only professional sport and mass media. Amateur sports dominate over professional sport in terms of number of people who engage in physical activity. Due to the development and wide-spread access to new digital technologies specially tailored for casual users, amateur sport is mediatized equally quickly, if not quicker, than professional sport, and its mediatization takes on many forms.[204]

The origins of analyzing the mediation of everyday life of "ordinary," physically active users, reach as far as the ancient world. If the main focus of interest lies in mediating human movement by the media, even walking can be perceived as an activity "mediated by the ancient technologies of shoes, pavements and pedestrian crossings."[205]

Contemporary physical activities are mediated and mediatized through di-verse technologies, resulting in humanistic and social reflection in the analy-sis of passers-by movement (e.g., "relationships of pedestrian-in-the-street and app-user-on-screen actions"[206]) or typologies resulting from mediatiza-tion (e.g., "iPod orchestrated walker"[207] or "contemporary mode of walking: together with touchscreen"[208]). Hitherto, in research located at the crossroads of media studies, ethnography and anthropology, the second course of trans-formation changes can be also noticed. For example, the concepts of "pe-destrianization and transformation of media"[209] prompts us to ask questions about the co-relation between transforming media technologies and processes mediated by them within the context of physical activity in which they are deployed. Physical activity, especially in the social dimension, generates changes in technology: modifications of the existing devices and applications and the emergence of new ones, and hybrid integration of technologies both at the material and virtual level.

Physical activity, further researched in this volume is understood "as any bodily movement produced by skeletal muscles that requires energy expenditure,"[210] intended and performed relatively regularly. Physical activ-ity encompasses a wide array of motion: from practicing specific, formally recognized sports (e.g., tennis), through alternative, informal disciplines (e.g., parkour), or those that fall within recreational activities (e.g., dancing), to everyday movement related to moving from place to place (e.g., cycling from home to work). The scope of physical activity also includes sports es-pecially predestined for mediatization, e.g., extreme sports (e.g., skydiving) or so-called lifestyle sports (e.g., surfing), which at times are based on the mediatization of the culture they generate. In those cases, media technologies such as digital cameras (invented for the needs of extreme sports, initially called sports cameras)[211] were used for the first time.

The mediatized world of physical activity is characterized by a large di-versity of the sub-worlds, both due to the richness of forms of activities and the media technologies deployed within their contexts. There is no doubt that all intended movement of the body using one's own muscles, performed relatively regularly during free time or associated with moving from place to place is an important element of everyday life, and its features are prone to the usage of media technologies. Currently, sport and physical activity are becoming increasingly fashionable,[212] which is supported by growing global economy, greater accessibility to relevant infrastructure, and increas-ing awareness of sports' impact on health, appearance, and well-being. As a result, amateur sport is becoming professionalized to a large extent while the infrastructure, commerce, and services related to physical activity expe-rience growth in line with that fashion. All this promotes innovation, and thus exposure to mediatization, resulting from media technologies becoming increasingly affordable (their prices are no longer excessive), infrastructure availability (mainly due to universal access to wireless Internet), and their convenience (technologies are increasingly handy (multi) functional, intuitive and aesthetically pleasing).

The diversification and dynamic development of media technologies and forms of activities lead to the heterogeneity of the mediatized physical activity. It is relatively easy to distinguish fans of particular disciplines, applying specific or diverse technologies in concrete or different sport disciplines. It can also be observed that certain forms of movement and types of technology fit together in a special way, thus creating specific sports-media worlds as they exhibit characteristic properties. Among them, we can observe mediatization mechanisms based on media saturation. Mediatization mechanisms may show differences deriving from the specificity of the sports-media world. It is therefore difficult to obtain a holistic, comprehensive picture of the physical activity mediatization as such since its variables are extremely diverse and rich.

On the other hand, it is possible to identify several dominating worlds, niche worlds, and intermediate worlds and, similarly, indicate technologies according to their popularity. This raises the question of the manner in which disciplines and technologies, which differ in terms of frequency of choice and application, correspond with each other. Also, it invites a discussion about the differences between the worlds emerging through the mechanisms of mediatization; the worlds shaped through practices at the individual (micro) level, leading to changes at the discipline or forming a new activity (mezzo) level and vice versa.

Similarly to studies examining other areas of everyday life, adapting a diachronic perspective on physical activity can be problematic. This is mainly due to the difficulties in accessing data,[213] which in the context of new technologies change rapidly. Therefore, synchronic approaches dominate, since they illustrate the as-is situation. Although studied situations are potentially very different from the preceding ones, even by only a few years, they are, to a limited extent, shaped by changes taking place over time. The challenge associated with that can be addressed when specific parameters (quantitative and qualitative) are applied in the research. Using them enables obtaining comparable results and, therefore, a detailed operationalization of parameters is necessary. Thus, research of the media saturation of physical activity is a step to form a new concept proposal and its operationalization in order to analyze the mediatization changes within a particular context, while potentially developing tools applicable in research of other spheres of everyday life.

In line with the chosen methodology of research on mediatization and to parameterize research on media saturation and on properties of physical activity, a specific research procedure and a set of methods has been adapted. Quantitative survey, used to explore mainly quantitative (to a lesser extent qualitative) aspects of media saturation, was carried out within a group of young, sporting and technologically active people. The obtained results illustrate how the degree, spectrum and other properties of technological and processual saturation are shaped. The analysis of collected statistical data was based on the proposed formulas to calculate saturation degree variations. The results of the research not only allowed for determining how the saturation of physical activity is shaped quantitatively, but were also used to distinguish sports-media dominant and niche worlds, and the initial diagnosis of the occurrence of desaturation. Furthermore, the results obtained were used for subsequent qualitative explorations.

NOTES

1. Mark B. Hansen, "Media Theory," *Theory, Culture & Society*, 23; 23 (2006): 297.
2. David Morley, "For a Materialist, Non–Media-centric Media Studies," *Television & New Media* 10.1 (2009): 114
3. Hansen, 297.
4. Marshall McLuhan: "The Medium is the Message," in *Understanding Media: The Extensions of Man* (New York: Signet, 1964), 23–35, 63–67.
5. Hansen, 298.
6. Simondon, Gilbert, *Du Mode des Objects Techniques* (Paris: Aubier, 1989) quoted in Mark B. Hansen (2006).
7. Nick Couldry and Andreas Hepp, *The Mediated Construction of Reality* (Polity: Cambridge, Malden, MA, 2017), 1.
8. Ibid., 2.
9. Ibid., 6.
10. Ibid., 7.
11. Ibid., 32.
12. Andreas Hepp, "Differentiation: Mediatization and Cultural Change," *Mediatization: Concept, Changes, Consequences*, ed. Knut Lundby (New York: Peter Lang, 2009), 140.
13. Look at Göran Bolin's translation and interpretation of Kjell Nowak's four types of mediatization and differentiation of "social interaction *within* as well as *with* and *through* (emphasis in original) 'the media environment'"; Göran Bolin, *Media Generations: Experience, Identity and Mediatised Social Change* (London and New York: Routledge, 2016): 23. More in Swedish: Kjell Nowak, "Medier Som Materiell och Mental Miljö," in *Medierna i Samhället: Igår, Idag, Imorgon*, ed. Ulla Carlsson (Göteborg: Nordicom 1996).
14. Couldry and Hepp, 31.
15. David Holmes, *Communication Theory: Media, Technology, Society* (Thousand Oaks: Sage Reference, 2005): 3. doi: http://dx.doi.org/10.4135/9781446220733.n1.

16. Couldry and Hepp, 29.

17. Noshir Contractor, Peter Monge, and Paul M. Leonardi, "Network Theory: Multidimensional Networks and the Dynamics of Sociomateriality: Bringing Technology Inside the Network," *International Journal of Communication* 5, 39 (2011): 684.

18. Wanda Orlikowski, "Using Technology and Constituting Structures: A Practice Lens for Studying Technology in Organisations," *Organisation Science* 11 (4) (2000): 404.

19. Paul M. Leonardi, "Digital Materiality? How Artifacts Without Matter, Matter," *First Monday* 15.6 (2010).

20. Niels Ole Finnemann, "Mediatization Theory and Digital Media," *Communications* 36 (2011): 83.

21. Ibid., 85.

22. Lynn Schofield Clark, "Mediatization: Concluding Thoughts and Challenges for the Future." In *Mediatized Worlds. Culture and Society in a Media Age*, eds. Andreas Hepp and Friedrich Krotz (Basingtoke: Palgrave Macmillan, 2014). 307–23: 309.

23. Leonardi, ibid.

24. Ibid.

25. Ibid.

26. Ibid.

27. Clark, 6.

28. Going beyond the perspective of a specific environment of one chosen medium is what J. Meyrowitz emphasizes (Joshua Meyrowitz, "Understandings of Media," *ETC: A Review of General Semantics* 56.1 (1999): 48; and looking from the perspective of integrated environment, A. Hepp, A. Breiter and U. Hasebrink specify that approach "a cross media approach"—"analysis how the various media come together in the communicative construction of social domains." Andreas Hepp, Andreas Breiter, and Uwe Hasebrink, "Rethinking Transforming Communication: An Introduction," in *Communicative Figurations, Transforming Communications—Studies in Cross-Media Research,* eds. Andreas Hepp, Andreas Breiter and Uwe Hasebrink (Cham: Palgrave McMillan 2016): 7.

29. Neil Postman, "The Reformed English Curriculum," in *High School 1980: The Shape of the Future in American Secondary Education*, ed. Alvin Eurich (New York: Pitman, 1970), 161.

30. Meyrowitz, 48.

31. Andreas Hepp, Andreas Breiter, and Uwe Hasebrink, 7.

32. Lance Strate, *Echoes and Reflections. On Media Ecology as a Field of Study* (Cresskill, NJ: Hampton Press, 2006), 17.

33. Mark Deuze, *Media Life* (Cambridge, MA: Polity, 2013), 3.

34. Luciano Floridi, "A Look into the Future Impact of ICT on our Lives," *The Information Society* 23 (2007): 4.

35. Christine Nystrom, "Towards a Science of Media Ecology: The Formulation of Integrated Conceptual Paradigms for the Study of Human Communication Systems" (Doctoral Dissertation, New York University, 1973), quoted after Strate, 18.

36. Strate, 101–02.

37. Finnemann, 80.

38. Roger Silverstone, "Why Study the Media?" (London: Sage Reference, 1999): 3. doi: http://dx.doi.org/10.4135/9781446219461.

39. Hansen, 299.

40. Deuze, XII–XIII.

41. Strate, 103.

42. Andreas Hepp, *Cultures of Mediatization* (Cambridge, MA: Polity, 2013), 97.

43. Nick Couldry, "Transvaluing Media Studies," *Media and Cultural Theory*, eds. James Curran and David Morley (Abingdon: Routledge, 2005): 190.

44. Ibid., 6.

45. David Morley, *Media, Modernity and Technology: The Geography of the New* (London: Routledge, 2007), 200.

46. Hepp, *Cultures Mediatization*, 133–34.

47. Couldry and Hepp, 34–35.

48. Friedrich Krotz, "Mediatization as a Mover in Modernity: Social and Cultural Change in the Context of Media Change," in *Mediatization of Communication. Handbooks of Communication Science* 21, ed. Knut Lundby (Berlin: De Gruyter Mouton, 2014): 137. Sonia Livingstone and Peter Lunt indicate three main areas of study on mediatization: system world (institutions of established power), civil society, and life-world; Sonia Livingstone and Peter Lunt, "Mediatization: an Emerging Paradigm for Media and Communication Studies," in *Mediatization of Communication. Handbooks of Communication Science* 21, ed. Knut Lundby (Berlin: De Gruyter Mouton, 2014): 716.

49. Couldry. *Mediatization or . . .*, 2008: 379.

50. The last of the terms is used most sporadically, e.g., Dan Lundberg, Krister Malm, and Owe Ronström, *Music, Media, Multiculture: Changing Musicscapes* (Svenskt visarkiv, 2003): 63, http://carkiv.musikverk.se/www/epublikationer/Lundberg_Malm_Ronstrom_Music_Media_Multiculture.pdf (retrieved online).

51. André Jansson and Magnus Andersson, "Mediatization at the Margins: Cosmopolitanism, Network Capital and Spatial Transformation in Rural Sweden," *Communications: The European Journal of Communication Research* 37(2) (2012): 178.

52. Couldry and Hepp, 17.

53. Ibid., 35.

54. Göran Bolin, "The Rhythm of Ages: Analyzing Mediatization Through the lens of Generations Across Cultures," *International Journal of Communication* (10) (2016): 5253.

55. Josef Pallas "Mediatization," in *The Sage Encyclopedia of Corporate Reputation*, ed. Craig E. Carroll (Thousand Oaks: Sage Reference, 2016), 445–48. doi: http://dx.doi.org/10.4135/9781483376493.n175, 3–4.

56. Bolin, "The Rythms . . .": 5253–54. Bolin, *Media Generations . . .*: 20–22.

57. Bolin, *Media Generations . . .*, 21.

58. Bolin, "The Rythms . . .": 5253–54.

59. Stig Hjarvard, "The Mediatization of Society. A Theory of the Media as Agents of Social and Cultural Change," *Nordicom Review* (2) (2008):105.

60. David Altheide, Rober Snow, *Media Logic* (Beverly Hills: Sage Publications 1979).

61. Hjarvard, 113.

62. Ibid.

63. Ibid. 114–15.

64. Friedrich Krotz and Andreas Hepp, "A Concretization of Mediatization: How Mediatization Works and Why 'Mediatized Worlds' are a Helpful Concept for Empirical Mediatization Research," in *Empedocles. European Journal for the Philosophy of Communication* 3 (2) (2013): 139.

65. Friedrich Krotz, "The Meta-process of Mediatization as a Conceptual Frame." *Global Media and Communication* 3 (3) (2007): 256.

66. Andreas Hepp, "Researching 'Mediatised Worlds': Non-mediacentric Media and Communication Research as a Challenge," in *Media and Communication Studies Interventions and Intersections,* eds. Nico Carpentier, Ilija Tomanić Trivundža, Pille Pruulmann-Vengerfeldt, Ebba Sundin, Tobias Olsson, Richard Kilborn, Hannu Nieminen, Bart Cammaerts (Tartu: Tartu University Press, 2010): 38.

67. Andreas Hepp, "Communicative Figurations. Researching Cultures of Mediatization," in *Media Practice and Everyday Agency in Europe*, eds. Leif Kramp, Nico Carpentier, Andreas Hepp, Ilija Tomanić Trivundža, Hannu Nieminen, Risto Kunelius, Tobias Olsson, Ebba Sundin and Richard Kilborn (Bremen: Edition Lumière, 2014): 88.

68. Hepp. "Researching 'Mediatised Worlds' . . ." 41–42.

69. Nick Couldry, "Digital Storytelling, Media Research and Democracy: Conceptual Choices and Alternative Futures," in *Digital Storytelling, Mediatized Stories: Self-representations in New Media. Digital Formations,* ed. Knut Lundby (New York: Peter Lang Publishing, 2008): 47.

70. Jean Baudrillard. *Symbolic Exchange and Death* (London: Sage Publications, 1993).

71. Livingstone and Lunt, 721.

72. Pallas, 3–5.

73. Couldry and Hepp, 53.

74. Deuze, XVI.

75. Couldry and Hepp, 192.

76. Hepp, Breiter, and Hasebrink, 6.

77. The theory of mediatization is currently going through a stage of intense development. The introduction to a book edited by Knut Lundby attempts to describe the stage of development of mediatization theory. The text shows paradigmatic diversification in the scope of problems and areas of mediatization. Knut Lundby, "Mediatization of Communication," in *Mediatization of Communication. Handbooks of Communication Science*, ed. Lundby Knut (Berlin: De Gruyter Mouton, 2014), 3–35.

78. Mirca Madianou and Daniel Miller, *Polymedia* (2010) http://blogs.nyu.edu/projects/materialworld/2010/09/polymedia.html, link does not exist (1.07.2018), quoted after Deuze, 56; "(. . .) we live our lives in a context of more, faster, all-encompassing, profoundly pervasive and therefore omnipresent media," Deuze, 132.

79. Tim O'Sullivan, Bryan Dutton, and Philip Rayner, "Studying the Media. An Introduction," (London: Edward Arnold, 1996): 3.

80. Clark, 4.

81. Charles Sanders Peirce, *Collected Papers of Charles Sanders Peirce* Vol. 5, eds. Charles Hortshorne and Paul Weiss (Cambridge: Harvard University Press, 1931–1958).

82. Mariusz Urbański, "O Rozumowaniach Abdukcyjnych," in *Propositiones*, eds. Tomasz Mróz and Mariusz Sieńko (Zielona Góra: Instytut Filozofii Uniwersytetu Zielonogórksiego, 2005), 143.

83. Urbański, 144. M. Urbański gives an example. Rule: All beans from this bag are white. The result: These beans are white. Condition: These beans are from this bag. Urbański, 144.

84. Urbański, 143.

85. Bartłomiej Skowron, philosopher in an interview with the author.

86. Clark, 4–5.

87. Urbański, 150.

88. Andreas Hepp and Friedrich Krotz, "Mediatized Worlds: Understanding Everyday Mediatization," in *Mediatized Worlds: Culture and Society in a Media Age*, eds. Andreas Hepp and Friedrich Krotz (London: Palgrave, 2014): 15.

89. Friedrich Krotz, *Neue Theorien Entwickeln. Eine Einführung in die Grounded Theory, die heuristische Sozialforschung und die Ethnographie anhand von Beispielen aus der Kommunikationsforschung* (Köln: Halem, 2005): 70; Friedrich Krotz, "Mediatisierung," *Fallstudien zum Wandel von Kommunikation* 84 (Wiesbaden: VS, 2007): 12, quoted by Hepp, *Cultures of Mediatization*, 48.

90. Hepp, 48.

91. Ibid.

92. Ibid., 49.

93. Ibid., 48.

94. Ibid., 127.

95. Barney G. Glaser and Anselm L. Strauss, *Discovery of Grounded Theory: Strategies for Qualitative Research* (New Brunswick, NJ: Aldine Transaction, 1967), 32.

96. Hepp, 130.

97. Ibid.

98. Ibid., 137.

99. Ibid., 139.

100. Louis Nicolas Vauquelin and G. L. Brismontier, *Dictionary of Chemistry: Containing the Principles and Modern Theories of the Science, with its Application to the Arts, Manufactures, and Medicine* (New York: G & C & Carvill, 1830), 406.

101. *Mosby's Medical Dictionary* (Liverport Lane: Elsevier, 2017), 1307.

102. Robert W. G. Hunt, "The Specification of Colour Appearance. I. Concepts and Terms," *Color Research & Application* 2(2) (1977): 55–68.

103. Christine Ammer and Dean S. Ammer, *Dictionary of Business and Economics* (New York, London: Macmillan, 1996), 413.

104. Pease, Roger W. Jr., *Merriam-Webster's Medical Dictionary* (Sprigfield, MA: Rebound by Sagebrush, 1995), 616.

105. Loran O'Bannon, *Dictionary of Ceramic Science and Engineering* (New York, London; Springer, 2012), 220.

106. Jay Newell, "Revisiting Schramm's Radiotown: Media Displacemenet and Saturation," *Journal of Radio Studies* 1 (2007): 6.

107. In the case of Todd Gitlin, the mentioned article dates back to the beginning of the twenty-first century.

108. Refers to the work of A. McRobbie; Newell, ibid.

109. Refers to the work of J. Baudrillard; Newell, ibid.

110. Refers to the work of T. Gitlin; Newell, ibid.

111. The terminology-related convergence between media saturation and social saturation, formulated by K. Gergen, has to be emphasized. Social saturation explains the phenomenon of shaping up social identity of an individual through diverse life-styles and visions of the world which takes place, e.g., through the use of so-called technology of social saturation. Kenneth J. Gergen, *The Saturated Self: Dilemmas of Identity in Contemporary Life* (New York: Basic Books, 1991).

112. David Holmes, *Communication Theory: Media, Technology, Society* (Thousand Oaks: Sage Reference, 2005): 3, doi: http://dx.doi.org/10.4135/9781446220733.n1.

113. Fausto Izcaray, *Mass Media Saturation Conditions and Information Gaps in Venezuela. Doctoral Dissertation* (Madison: University of Wisconsin, 1980), quoted after Newell, 6.

114. John, L. Sherry, "Media Saturation and Entertainment-education," *Communication Theory* 2 (2002): 208.

115. Newell, 6.

116. This applies both to his work from 2007 and 2008.

117. Jay Newell, Joseph, J. Pilotta, John, C. Thomas, "Mass Media Displacement and Saturation," *The International Journal on Media Management* 4 (2008), 131.

118. Gitlin, 142. Moreover, while writing about the exposal, T. Gitlin focuses mainly on the flow of images and sounds reaching the recipient through various technologies and not on the properties of those technologies.

119. Deuze, X. Examining media saturation is a response to the question once asked by Ien Ang: "what it means, or *what it is like* (emphasis in original), to live in a media-saturated world"; Ien Ang, *Living Room Wars. Rethinking Media Audiences* (London: Routledge, 1995), 72.

120. Devereux Eoin, *Understanding the Media* (London: Sage Publications, 2007). It seems quite symptomatic that media saturation is indicated in the first chapter of the textbook as a key issue, alongside mass media, to name only a few, but without formulating any definition. A similar situation refers to media studies monographs. In a book titled *Digital Journalism* Janet Jones and Lee Salter discuss the influence of "media saturation and diffusion of attention" on the size of the audience and the quality of content in local services, however, they do not explain what they mean by that term; Janet Jones and Lee Salter, *Digital Journalism* (Thousand Oaks: Sage Reference, 2012): 13. doi: http://dx.doi.org/10.4135/9781446288634.n6.

121. Nick Couldry, "Mediatization or Mediation? Alternative Understandings of the Emergent Space of Digital Storytelling," *New Media & Society* 3 (2008): 380.

122. Specified then by N. Couldry after R. Silverston as mediation; Roger Silverstone, "Complicity and Collision in the Mediation of Everyday Life," *New Literary History* 4 (2002): 761.

123. O'Sullivan, Dutton, and Rayner, 3 and 8.

124. Bogusława Dobek-Ostrowska, *Komunikowanie Polityczne i Publiczne* (Warszawa" Państwowe Wydawnictwo Naukowe PWN, 2007), 276.

125. O'Sullivan, Dutton, and Rayner, 272.

126. Dobek-Ostrowska, 157. Unfortunately, a closer definition of what constitutes of "saturation degree" and how it can be used has not been offered.

127. O'Sullivan, Dutton, and Rayner, 1.

128. "In other words, what appears to be 'postmodern' is simply an elevated form of media saturation and consumerism reserved for those first world individuals who can afford such a lifestyle." Andy Bennett, "Postmodernism," in Andy Bennet, *Culture and Everyday Life* (Thousand Oaks: Sage Reference, 2005): 16, doi: http://dx.doi.org/10.4135/9781446219256.n2.

129. I.e., Renata Rusin-Dybalska, "Nowy Wymiar Komunikowania Politycznego na Przykładzie Języka Prezydenta Czech Miloša Zemana," *Rozprawy Komisji Językowej ŁTN* Z. 62 (2016): 117.

130. "On average, people in the United States spend one third of their lives immersed in media, whether this takes the form of watching television, film, or videos; listening to music; reading print magazines and books; or surfing on the Internet. Given this media saturation, it is important to explore the tools needed to effectively navigate these media (. . .)." Ernest Morrell, "Media Literacy," in *Encyclopedia of African Amercian Education*, ed. Kofi Lomotey (Thousand Oaks: Sage Reference: 2010): 2, doi: http://dx.doi.org/10.4135/9781412971966.n158.

131. "Opportunities for media consumption have expanded dramatically since then with the advent of new technologies—first television and then the Internet. Some claim that society suffers from media saturation and that the media dominate our experience of the world." John L. Sullivan, "Mass Consumption," in *The Sage Glossary of the Social and Behavioral Sciences*, ed. John L. Sullivan (Thousand Oaks: Sage Reference, 2009): 2, doi: http://dx.doi.org/10.4135/9781412972024.n1540.

132. Couldry and Hepp, 55.

133. Although A. Hepp does not define saturation, he notices the diversification of media in various areas and the saturation *degree* corresponding to them through that media; Hepp, 68.

134. Friedrich Krotz and Andreas Hepp, "A Concretization of Mediatization: How Mediatization Works and Why 'Mediatized Worlds' are a Helpful Concept for Empirical Mediatization Research," in *Empedocles. European Journal for the Philosophy of Communication* 3 (2) (2013): 139.

135. Knut Lundby, "Mediatization of Communication,," 20.

136. Lundby, 20.

137. Kopecka-Piech, Katarzyna, "Media Saturation as a Techno-social Phenomenon. Selected Examples of Smartphonisation in Social Life," in: Studia Kulturoznawcze 3 (2017): 101.

138. See Introduction.

139. Kopecka-Piech, "Media Saturation as a Techno-social Phenomenon," 101

140. W. Orlikowski assumes that after Giddens; Anthony Giddens, *The Constitution of Society: Outline of the Theory of Structuration* (Berkeley: University of California Press, 1984); Orlikowski, 406.

141. By "the everyday life-world" I understand, after Schutz and Luckmann, "the region of reality in which man can engage himself"; Alfred Schutz and Thomas Luckmann, *The Structures of the Life World* (Evanston, IL: Northwestern University Press, 1973), 3.

142. Roger Silverstone, "The Sociology of Mediation and Communication," in *The International Handbook of Sociology*, eds. Craig Calhoun, Chris Rojek, and Bryan Turner (London: Sage Publications, 2000), 189.

143. "Human expressivity is capable of objectivation, that is, it manifests itself in products of human activity that are available both to their producers and to other men as elements of a common world. Such objectivations serve as more or less enduring indices of the subjective processes of their producers, allowing their availability to extend beyond the face-to-face situation in which they can be directly apprehended," Peter L. Berger and Thomas Luckmann, *The Social Construction of Reality: A Treatise in the Sociology of Knowledge* (London: Penguin, 1996), 49.

144. "Reification is the apprehension of human phenomena as if they were things, that is, in non-human or possibly suprahuman terms. Another way of saying this is that reification is the apprehension of the products of human activity as if they were something other than human products–such as facts of nature, results of cosmic laws, or manifestations of divine will," Berger and Luckmann, 106.

145. "'Resources of meaning' here means 'media products' such as 'text,' 'film' or 'website' to which we relate when we generate meaning in (media) communication"; Hepp, 70.

146. Ibid.

147. Gregor McLennan, "Post-Marxism and the 'Four Sins' of Modernist Theorizing," *New Left Review* (218) 53 (1996): 66–67.

148. Knut Lundby, "Notes on Interaction and Mediatization," in *Media Practice and Everyday Agency in Europe*, eds. Leif Kramp, Leif Kramp, Nico Carpentier, Andreas Hepp, Ilija Tomanić Trivundža, Hannu Nieminen, Risto Kunelius, Tobias Olsson, Ebba Sundin, and Richard Kilborn (Bremen: Edition Lumière, 2014), 42.

149. Ibid.

150. Pitirim A. Sorokin, *Society, Culture, and Personality, Their Structure and Dynamics* (New York, London: Harper & Brothers Publishers, 1947), 52–53.

151. Ibid., 53.

152. Ibid.

153. Ibid.

154. Ibid., 52.

155. Lundby, 42.

156. Lundby, 50.

157. The discursive dimension of mediatization is based on the material properties of technology. "The practical and material characteristics of media systems and technologies shape what can be thought and expressed," Norm Friesen and Theo Hug, "The Mediatic Turn: Exploring Concepts for Media Pedagogy," in *Mediatization: Concept, Changes, Consequences*, ed. Knut Lundby (Frankfurt a. M.: Peter Lang, 2009), 67.

158. Hepp, *Cultures of Mediatization*, 57.

159. Ibid., 68.

160. Johan Fornäs, "Media Times. The Mediatization of Third-Time Tools: Culturalizing and Historicizing Temporality," *International Journal of Communication* 10 (2016): 5222.

161. Proposed formulas to calculate the degree of saturation can be found in chapter 2.

162. Friedrich Krotz, *Mediatisierung. Fallstudien zum Wandel von Kommunikatio* (Wiesbaden: VS, 2007), 37–43, quoted after Hepp, Cultures of Mediatization, 52–53.

163. Couldry and Hepp, 39.

164. Ibid., 56.

165. Ibid., 142. The authors refer to the statements by Evgeny Morozov; Evgeny Morozov, "El Derecho a Desconectarse," *El Pais* (2015); and Gilles Deleuze; Gilles Deleuze, *Negotiations* 1972–1990 (New York: Columbia University Press, 1995).

166. Deuze, *Media Life*, XIII.

167. Ibid., X.

168. The best example of such people is those who suffer from electromagnetic hypersensitivity. Caitlin Dewey, "Are 'WiFi Allergies' a Real Thing? A Quick Guide to Electromagnetic Hypersensitivity," *The Washington Post* (2015) (retrieved online).

169. Hartmut Rosa, *Social Acceleration: A New Theory of Modernity* (New York: Columbia University Press, 2013).

170. Couldry and Hepp, 216.

171. Andreas Hepp and Uwe Hasebrink, "Researching Transforming Communications in Times of Deep Mediatization: A Figurational Approach," *Communicative Figurations, Transforming Communications—Studies in Cross-Media Research*, eds. Andreas Hepp, Andreas Breiter, Uwe Hasebrink (Cham: Palgrave Macmillan, 2018), 18.

172. Fornäs, 5221.

173. Stig Hjarvard, *The Mediatization of Culture and Society* (London: Routledge, 2013), 155.

174. Fornäs, 5222.

175. Ibid., 5221.

176. Roger Silverstone, "The Sociology of Mediation and Communication," *The Sage Handbook of Sociology*, eds. Craig Calhoun, Chris Rojek, and Bryan Turner (London: Sage Reference, 2015), 16. doi: http://dx.doi.org/10.4135/9781848608115.n11.

177. In order to cut off from the mobile telecommunication's electromagnetic waves, people install insulating nets in the windows of their homes or detectors of approaching drones on their fences.

178. Marian Adolf, "Clarifying Mediatization: Sorting Through a Current Debate," *Empedocles: European Journal for the Philosophy of Communication* 3.2 (2011): 154.

179. Deuze, X.

180. Ibid., XI.

181. More on desaturation can be found in chapter 5.

182. Deuze, 79.

183. Pallas, 4.

184. Friedrich Krotz, "From a Social Worlds Perspective to the Analysis of Mediatized Worlds," in *Media Practice and Everyday Agency in Europe*, eds. Leif Kramp, Leif Kramp, Nico Carpentier, Andreas Hepp, Ilija Tomanić Trivundža, Hannu Nieminen, Risto Kunelius, Tobias Olsson, Ebba Sundin, and Richard Kilborn (Bremen: Edition Lumière, 2014): 70.

185. Hepp, "Differentiation: Mediatization and Cultural Change," 150; Hepp and Hasebring, 16.

186. Krotz and Hepp, 18.

187. Ibid., 19.

188. Friesen and Hug, 3.

189. Krotz and Hepp, 20–21.

190. Clark, 3.

191. Couldry and Hepp, 20.

192. Strauss, Anselm, "A Social World Perspective," *Studies in Symbolic Interaction* 1.1 (1978): 119–128.

193. Hepp, *Cultures of Mediatization*, 92.

194. Ibid., 83.

195. See, e.g., David Rowe, "Global Media Sport: Flows, Forms and Futures," in *Sport, Media and Mega-events.* eds. Lawrence A. Wenner and Andrew C. Billings (London: Taylor & Francis, 2017).

196. Kirsten Frandsen, "Mediated (Dis)Contuinities: Contesting Pasts, Presents and Futures," (Conference Discussion, 6th European Communication Conference, ECREA Prague, November 11, 2016).

197. Brett Hutchins and David Rowe, "From Broadcast Rationing to Digital Plenitude; The Changing Dynamics of the Media Sport Content Economy," *Television and New Media* (4) (2009): 355.

198. David Rowe, *Sport, Culture, and The Media: The Unruly Trinity* (Maidenhead: McGraw-Hill Education, 2003): 4.

199. Kirsten Frandsen, "Mediatization of Sports," in *Mediatization of Communication*, ed. Knut Lundby (Berlin: Mouton de Gruyter, 2014).

200. Kirsten Frandsen, "Sports Broadcasting, Journalism and the Challenge of New Media." *MedieKultur: Journal of Media and Communication Research* 28 (53) (2012).

201. Kirsten Frandsen, *Tour de France: Mediatization of Sport and Place*, in *Sport, Media and Mega-events*, eds. Lawrence A. Wenner, Andrew C. Billings (New York: Routledge, 2017).

202. Kirsten Frandsen, "Sports Organizations in a New Wave of Mediatization," *Communication & Sport* 4 (4) (2016).

203. Stine Lomborg and Kirsten Frandsen. "Self-tracking as Communication," *Information, Communication & Society* 19.7 (2016): 1015–27.

204. Brett Hutchins and David Rowe, *Sport beyond Television: The Internet, Digital Media and the Rise of Networked Media Sport*, eds. Brett Hutchins and David Rowe, Vol. 40 (New York: Routledge, 2012); Marcos Dias, "The Converging Worlds of 'Surfing the Web' and the Sport of Surfing" in *A Scholarly Affair: Proceedings of the Cultural Studies Association of Australasia 2010 National Conference*, eds. Baden Offord and Rob Garbutt (Lismore: Centre for Peace and Social Justice and the School of Arts and Social Science, 2011) (retrieved online); Clifton Evers, "Masculinity, Sport and Mobile Phones," in *The Routledge Companion to Mobile Media*, eds. Gerard Goggin and Larissa Hjorth (London and New York: Routledge, 2014): 375–84; Paul Gilchrist and Belinda Wheaton, "New Media Technologies in Lifestyle Sport," in *Digital Media Sport: Technology, Power and Culture in the Network Society*, eds. Brett Hutchins and David Rowe (New York: Routledge, 2013), 169–87. Glen Thompson, *From the Water to the Web: Surfing, Self, and the New Media in South Africa* (2013) (retrieved online); Holly Thorpe, *Transnational Mobilities in Action Sport Cultures* (Basingstoke: Palgrave Macmillan, 2014).

205. Eric Laurier, Barry Brown, and Moira McGregor, "Mediated Pedestrian Mobility: Walking and the Map App," *Mobilities* 11(1) (2016): 118.

206. Ibid., 117.

207. Term proposed by Laurier, E., Brown, and McGregor, B., to describe phenomenon observed by Michael Bull. Laurier, Brown, and McGregor, 14. More in Michael Bull, "The World According to Sound Investigating the World of Walkman Users," *New Media & Society* 3 (2) (2001): 179–97; Michael Bull, "No Dead Air! The iPod and the Culture of Mobile Listening," *Leisure Studies* 24 (4) (2005), 343–55.

208. Laurier, Brown, and McGregor, 16.

209. Ibid., 4.

210. WHO, *Physical Activity* (n.d.) (retrieved online).

211. Laurier, Brown, and McGregor, 5.

212. "The increasing need to become physically fit, and furthermore, to share that show their progress, has become a trend, and for some even a lifestyle," Amanda DiFonzo, *Cyberbullying, Social Media & Fitness Selfies: An Evolutionary Perspective*. Master Thesis (Ontario: Brock University St. Catharines, 2016), 3.

213. Andreas Hepp, Stig Hjarvard and Knut Lundby, "Mediatization: Theorizing the Interplay between Media, Culture and Society," *Media, Culture & Society* 37(2) (2015): 320.

Chapter Two

Media Saturation
and Physical Activity

Quantitative Approaches

According to the methodology outlined in chapter 1, it was decided to adopt a tailored research procedure and a set of methods positioned within the context of media saturation and physical activity. Therefore, quantitative survey was conducted among a group of young, physically active, and technologically savvy people. The obtained results illustrate the interplay between the degree, spectrum, and other properties of technological and processual saturation and their subsequent development and shaping. The analysis of collected statistical data was primarily based on the proposed calculation formulas applied to gauge saturation degree variants. The results of the research not only allowed for determining the shaping precedent of physical activity saturation in a quantitative manner, but were also used to distinguish sports-media dominant and niche worlds, and the initial examination of the desaturation occurrence. Finally, the obtained results were used for further qualitative explorations.

METHODOLOGY

The research carried out in the first phase had two goals. Firstly, the survey served as a test of the tools designed for media saturation measurement. Secondly, it allowed to specify selected qualitative and quantitative aspects of media saturation in physical activity among a chosen group of respondents.

The primary aim of the empirical research was to obtain a general insight of the spectrum, degree, and quality specification of the media saturation in physical activity among sporty and technologically savvy participants with the use of a new research tool. The secondary aim was to obtain data directing further qualitative research with the use of in-depth, semi-structured interviews, and observations, to name just a few methods. The objective was to develop a deeper understanding of the sport-media worlds in the surveyed cohort and to carry out an in-depth characteristic of saturation analysis in the selected areas.

The research subject focused on the media technologies used during physical activity, the mediated processes realized in that activity, and, to a limited extent, the media content created within.

The application of thirty-two technologies, the occurrence of twenty-two processes and the creation of sports media content for the fifteen forms of movement (most popular and niche forms of movement, referred to as "others") were studied.[1]

The surveyed group were young individuals (aged between 15 and 24), living in large European urban agglomeration (Wrocław, Poland), comprising of 286 physically active people (at least 60 minutes per week) of whom the majority declared using media technologies during physical activity (286 out of 300).

The first research query was concerned with the following problem: what is the spectrum and the degree of media saturation in physical activity among the surveyed group? In other words, the aim was to answer the following questions:

- What media technologies are used during physical activity?
- What are their functions and how are they applied?
- What processes are mediated by those technologies?
- What are the relationships between the deployed technologies and different forms of physical activity in which participants engaged?

The second query pertained to the respondents' opinion on the meaning of the media saturation of physical activity. The aim was to answer the following questions:

- What are the reasons for media technologies use in physical activity?
- How does media technology influence physical activity?
- What implications of media saturation in physical activity have been observed and—potentially—how are they evaluated?

The answers to the above questions enabled researchers to identify quantitative and qualitative aspects of technological and processual saturation. For example, they allow for measuring the variants of technological and processual saturation. To this end, new calculation formulae were introduced. Using the data obtained in the survey, calculations were made according to the newly proposed degree formulae: the degree of individual technological/ processual saturation (ITS/IPS), the degree of technological/processual saturation in the surveyed sample (TSS/PSS), and the degree of technological/ processual saturation of a particular form of physical activity in the surveyed sample (TSFS/PSPF). The obtained data also allowed to characterize the basic qualitative aspects of technological saturation, including the functions of media technologies used in physical activity and a chosen mediated process (mainly communicating the content about physical activity). While obtained data allowed for determining the particular features of media saturation of physical activity, directions for further research have also been established.

The research involved distributing a traditional questionnaire at schools, student associations, and sport clubs,[2] with respondents confirming their age and residency prior to the completion of questionnaires. Out of 300 attempted questionnaires, 297 were subject to analysis; incomplete questionnaires were eliminated (particularly those missing respondents' age, address, and those outside of the sample geographical boundaries or insufficient frequency of physical activity engagement), as well as those demonstrating discrepancies that indicated accidental responses. The analysis of saturation with the particular media technologies was carried out based on 286 questionnaires since 14 respondents declared absence of engagement with media technologies during physical activity.

The choice of the surveyed population was dictated by results of desktop research on existing data.[3] It was assumed that the survey population should be selected on the basis of research conducted hitherto—a group in which survey of media saturation would result with the widest and most comprehensive characteristics of the problem and thus providing the most substantial opportunity to show the complexity and variedness of the phenomenon as well as offering a wide range of possibilities for further exploration of survey areas, including sport-media worlds of particular forms of physical activity representatives or the worlds of physically active users of particular media technologies.

The most recent statistical research available in Poland (commissioned by commercial and public institutions) concerning both physical activity and the use of new technologies, including the Internet, was used. This led to the selection of young people living in a large city as the surveyed population. The research shows that young people living in large agglomerations are both the most physically active and the most involved in the application of technology (also due to access to it, e.g., to the Internet) and open to the effects of their rapid development.[4]

The chosen population was aged between 18 and 24 and living in Wrocław Agglomeration as the most promising in terms of the possibility to grasp the quantitative and qualitative diversity of the researched phenomenon. Wrocław is a large Polish city, which, according to existing research, means higher involvement in physical activity and better access to technologies, e.g., the Internet. It was decided to include in the survey sample individuals who live not only in cities but in agglomerations due to the growing urban, demographic, and administrative importance of the adjacent municipalities; all respondents went to school, studied in colleges, or worked in a city. The geographical location of Wrocław (on the plain, but not far from the mountains, and lakes, slightly larger than the sea) and in the temperate climate zone also offers the possibility of practicing various forms of movement, both indoor and outdoor; both summer, winter, and year-round sports.

This choice also allowed for capturing the formative years of youth, when experience, including media experience, is shaped and it imprints on later experiences with the "grammar" affecting all subsequent experiences, including the learning and perception of media.[5] The researched sample included a group of very young people,[6] aged between 15 and 17 years who are seldom targeted in surveys.[7] The rationale for this population sample age extension was dictated by the need to compare the behavior and experience of very young people (school age) and young people (university age). The survey cohort constructed that way also allowed for establishing the advancement of media saturation depending on the age of technology users and specifying shape of the leading mediatization changes which may come later in larger scale.[8]

Although the sample was purposeful rather than random, the research allowed for effective testing of the saturation research method and obtaining results whose representativeness for the studied population is highly probable. This population is very specific (young people living in the Wrocław agglomeration, regularly physically active, using media technologies during training). In a randomly selected sample of the above parameters, the level of trust of 91 percent, with the error margin of 0.5[9] would be obtained. However, these data should be treated as a starting point for further research. They allowed to test new saturation calculation formulas and, first of all, to recognize the area of physical activity of young people, thus directing the qualitative research.

The survey included twenty-six closed questions with one answer, multiple choice questions, and rankings. Based on the desktop research on the existing data on physical activity and based on initial research and observations, the questionnaire included the list of media technologies, forms of physical activity, functions of technologies, and the implications of their usage.

At the same time, the usage of thirty-two media technologies was checked against fifteen forms of physical activity and twenty-two mediatized processes that take place during physical activity.

With regard to technology: It might be called "media matrix" as it is a set of media technologies available at a certain time and place.[10] It is worth emphasizing the functional inseparability of the particular technologies that were subject to the survey. Some technologies are not separable in practice and they were not divided in line with the opposition: first-order media—second-order media.

> For Kubicek, 'first-order media' are technological systems with particular functions and potentialities for the dissemination of information in its technical sense, i.e., the Internet as a vehicle for the Transmission Control Protocol/Internet Protocol (TCP/IP) model. 'Second-order media' are in addition socio-cultural institutions of communication. This would be, for example, not the Internet itself but an online newspaper or email.[11]

Specification of the list of technologies was not dictated by the priority of separability, but by the potential of each of the technology to constitute of a separate, distinguishable media technology with specific characteristics that can decide about creating a particular media and sport world. Despite the inseparability of categories, in practice that means that some of them can fit in others (e.g., a mobile application in a smartphone) due to constructing adequate questions and obtaining responses to them, calculations were carried out to allow for the measurement of the degree of technology saturation precisely in the surveyed cohort. The principal goal of the first stage of the research was also achieved: sport-media worlds were isolated and subjected to further research. Similarly, inseparable typology of technologies (in this case, self-tracking technologies) can be found in other research (e.g., physical devices, apps, exergames, and web apps are distinguished).[12]

Separate questions were devoted to the process of communication, e.g., creating, publishing, and receiving media content about physical activity. The survey included seventeen functions of media technologies and seven main implications of their usage.

SURVEY RESULTS

The presentation of basic survey arrangements will be followed by test results on technological saturation and processual saturation, with the division of saturation aspects into quantitative and qualitative.

Basic Arrangements

Men dominated among the respondents comprising of almost 56 percent of the sample. The research included individuals aged between 15 and 24, however a larger category was made up by participants between the ages of 20 and 24 (61.2%) than 15- to 19-year-olds (38.8%). The educational background of the respondents is varied and related to their age. The largest group (45.6%) are respondents with post middle-school education (e.g., high school or vocational) followed by those with higher education (28.2%) and middle school (24.1%). People with primary education comprised of only 2 percent of the surveyed respondents. Based on the responses it can be stated that 97 percent of surveyed participants take up physical activity lasting at least sixty minutes per week on a regular basis. Men take up physical activity more often than women (98.8% and 94.7%, respectively). However, that discrepancy is very slight.

The most common form of physical activity is gym-based exercising and running, as indicated by more than half of the physically active respondents. This is followed by cycling (one-third of the respondents), and exercising at home (one-quarter of surveyed respondents). More than 20 percent of respondents declare that they play team sports such as football or volleyball. The diversity of forms of physical activities is non-uniform among the surveyed respondents; some of them declare one activity whereas others listed up to a dozen activities. After equating those results, it can be stated that, on average, the respondents regularly take up three different forms of physical activities. Figure 2.1 shows a detailed breakdown of those results.

Among other sports the respondents listed: badminton (6), tennis (5), cross-fit (4), hand ball (3), horse riding (3), yoga (3), squash (3), acrobatics (2), climbing (2), parkour (2), shooting sports (2), windsurfing (2), kitesurfing (1), bowling (1), golf (1), track and field (1), and fencing (1).

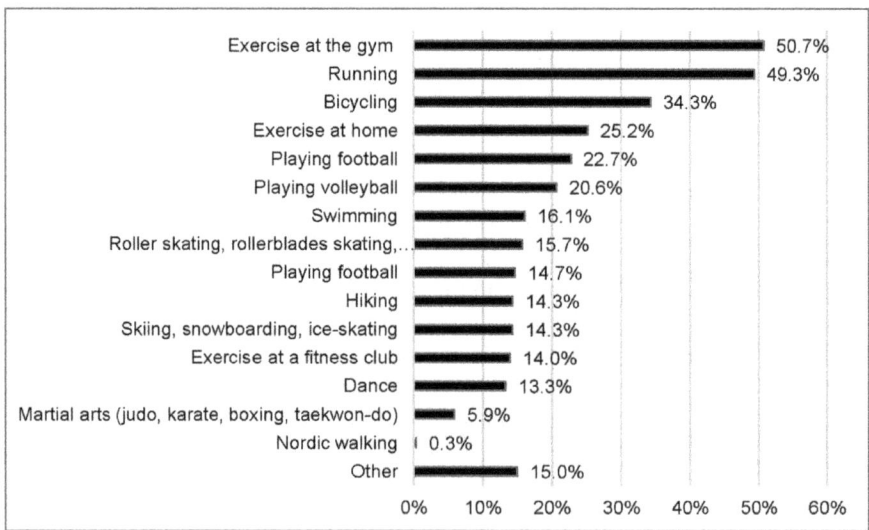

Figure 2.1. Question: Which of the activities do you take up at least once a week and not less than sixty minutes per week? (N=286)

Source: Survey data. The percentage in the graph exceeds 100 since the participants could choose more than one response.

The correlation of survey results pertaining to particular forms of physical activities preferred by men and women shows significant differences. Men exercise at the gym definitely more often (61.3 percent of men compared with 38.2 percent of women) and play football (34.4 percent of men vs. 7.3 percent of women); this trend is also apparent in swimming and basketball. Women definitely more often exercise at home than men (35.8 percent of women compared to 16.9 percent of men), they take up classes in fitness clubs (25.2 percent of women vs. 4.4 percent of men), dance (22.8 percent of women vs. 6.3 percent of men) and they rollerblade, roller skate, and skateboard more often.

Media Saturation of Physical Activity—Quantitative Aspects

The Spectrum and the Degree of Technological Saturation

By a spectrum we should understand the scope of technologies and mediatized processes specified based on the existing data or initial survey, which are used in a particular time and place during a particular activity, and which can undergo detailed survey. In accordance with the adopted definition, the research investigated what media technologies are used during physical activity of the respondents. Moreover, the typologies of the technologies were isolated and alternative variants of the degree of technological saturation were specified and calculated.

The Spectrum

As the survey results show, the spectrum of media technologies used during physical activity is very broad.

The basic typologies of media technologies distinguished in the research are:

- first-order technologies (e.g., devices) and second-order technologies (e.g., applications);
- universal technologies (e.g., smartphones) and technologies dedicated to physical activities (e.g., Endomondo mobile application);
- interactive, engaging technologies (e.g., messengers) and accompanying technologies (e.g., radio);
- traditional technologies (so-called mass media, e.g., television) and new media technologies (digital, interactive, e.g., kinetic-type games);
- wearable technologies (e.g., smartwatches) and body-external technologies (e.g., simulators); and
- stationary technologies (e.g., traditional radio sets) and mobile technologies (e.g., smartwatches).

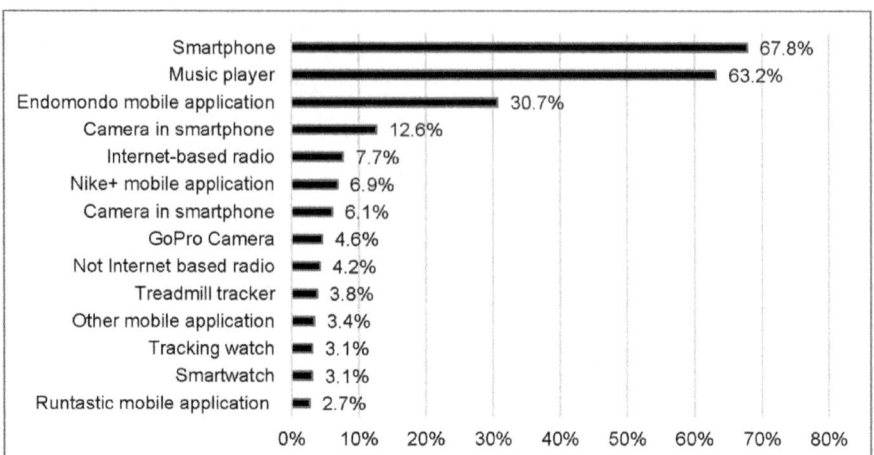

Figure 2.2. This graph illustrates the technologies participants deployed during physical activity. (N=261).

Source: Survey data. The percentage in the graph exceeds 100 since the participants could choose more than one response.

While the range of the responses was diverse, a vast majority of technologies is used only by a small percentage of respondents. Among thirty-one analyzed technologies, only four are used by more than 10 percent of active respondents, and fifteen technologies are used by less than two percent of surveyed people and thus they can be considered as niche technologies. New, digital technologies dominate: they comprise of twelve out of fourteen technologies used during physical activity by at least 2 percent of the survey's participants.

Smartphone is the technology used during physical activity by the highest percentage of respondents (67.8%). It is hybrid, converged technology that facilitates the usage of a variety of media of the second-order; it can function as an interactive, engaging medium (e.g., messenger) and accompanying medium (e.g., music player). Due to the design allowing for many technologies to be built into smartphones and to connect with many accessories (headphones, speakers, microphone, etc.), it is possible to expand the number of its functionalities; they can be used in many activities.

Fewer users (63.2%) use personal music players during physical activity. For the purpose of this study, the music player is understood as both individual devices specialized for listening to music (mp3, mp4, iPod, and other portable devices) as well as music applications for smartphones. The research revealed that 27.8 percent of individuals use a smartphone to listen to music during physical activity. It is worth noting that both of those dominating technologies are universally used across both age groups.

Similarly, while used less often, camera and video camera are also applied in a universal manner. They are used not only in physical activity, but saturate everyday life in different areas, too. Every eighth respondent uses a smartphone camera during physical activity and every sixteenth respondent uses a smartphone video camera. In the group of technologies used to document physical activity, GoPro-type video camera was also present, although on a much lower popularity scale (4.6%).

Among technologies designed for people who are physically active, respondents most often listed two mobile applications: Endomondo (30.7%) and Nike+ (6.9%). Those were followed by Runtastic (2.7%), SHealth (three people), Tabata Timer, Sports Tracker, Run the Map, MyFitnessPal, Gym Run, Adi Coach, Strava, Google Fit, Run Keeper (listed by singular respondents).

Low level of usage was declared for Nike+ (6.9%) as well as accompanying media, such as Internet radio (7.7%) and regular radio (4.2%).

The following technologies showed a completely niche character, both in terms of participating in the entire group of technologies used (below 1%), and the percentage of their users (below 2%):

• traditional media technologies: TV and film and their digital counterparts (Internet TV, VOD, DVD, film streaming),
• advanced and specialist technologies (tracker-band, sensors, augmented reality, Kinect-type games, drones),
• cameras and video cameras that are not integrated with a smartphone or do not belong to the category of portable mini-cameras such as GoPro.

Due to the wide spectrum of technologies and a multitude of forms of physical activity, the variety of media worlds in which participants engage is extensive. Different technologies are commonly used for certain forms of physical activity and some of those forms are clearly more popular than others. For that reason, it is appropriate to differentiate between sport-media worlds that are popular ("mass") in character and niche. The highly individualized use of the technologies is further assisted by their numerous combinations shared between various forms of physical activity. On the one hand, this allows for specific patterns of mediatization to emerge within the context of newly constructed realities of popular sport disciplines and technologies. On the other hand, separate, unique and particular sport-media worlds as well as those of niche technologies and disciplines can be researched. Finally, there are also special worlds, generated through the connection of particular sport disciplines and technologies that align and interconnect in a particular manner.

Variants of the Degree of Technological Saturation

In order to specify the quantitative degree of media saturation in the researched sample, the following alternatives of saturation measurement were proposed:

- the degree of individual technological saturation (ITS): the number of technologies used by a person (according to the questionnaire declaration) divided by the number of all technologies used by the respondents in the surveyed sample (at least one of the respondents had to indicate the technology in question in order for it to be recognized) multiplied by 100 percent,

ITS = number of technologies used by a person ÷ number of all used technologies · 100 percent

- the degree of technological saturation in the surveyed sample (TSS): the average number of technologies used by the respondents divided by the number of all technologies used by the respondents in the surveyed sample multiplied by 100 percent,

TSS = average number of used technologies ÷ number of all used technologies · 100 percent

- the degree of technological saturation of a particular form of physical activity in the surveyed sample (TSFS): the average number of technologies used by the respondents divided by the number of all technologies used by the respondents who engage in particular forms of physical activity in the surveyed sample multiplied by 100 percent.

TSFS = average number of used technologies ÷ the number of all technologies used in a particular form of physical activity · 100 percent

The calculations of the technological saturation show the number technologies used during a physical activity. They also show the degree to which the available options are utilized, allowing to specify the absorptiveness of the particular activity by media technologies, and assess to what extent the multiple technologies are used simultaneously.

Based on the measurement of the first variant of the degree of technological saturation (ITS), it is possible to indicate minimum and maximum results obtained by the particular respondents. It allows for drawing comparisons within the surveyed sample[13] which enables a deeper explanation of the mechanisms of mediatization.[14]

The third variant of the degree of saturation may be applied in a similar manner: the relative degree of technological saturation of a given form of physical activity in the surveyed sample (TSFS) enables observation of particular forms of physical activity in the entire sample and their comparison.[15]

The Results of Calculations

Table 2.1.   Variants of degree of technological saturation

The degree of individual technological saturation (ITS)	The degree of technological saturation of the surveyed group (TSS)	Relative degree of technological saturation of a particular form of physical activity in the surveyed sample (TSFS)
ITS min.: $1 \div 31 \cdot 100\% = 3.226\%$ ITS max.: $7 \div 31 \cdot 100\% = 22.58\%$	TSS: $2.4 \div 31 \cdot 100\%$ $= 7.742\%$	TSFS running: $2.57 \div 31 \cdot 100\% = 8.290\%$ TSFS gym: $2.21 \div 31 \cdot 100\% = 7.129\%$

Source: Own calculations based on survey data.

The results obtained in the surveyed sample show that TSS amounts to 7.742 percent, which may seem a low number. The majority of technologies from the available spectrum is not applicable. On average, 2.4 media technologies are used during physical activity, which demonstrates a lack of need for the integration of multiple technologies and a rather simplified model of functioning with the technology.

The maximum ITS and TSS are relatively low (only 22.58 percent and 7.742 percent, respectively), which confirms the nondominating character of most of the surveyed media technologies. The calculations of TSFS for the most popular forms of activity show that the degree of the use of available technologies range in these forms of activity is close to average; in terms of running, it exceeds the average by 0.5 percent, and in the case of gym workouts, it is about 0.5 percent lower than the average. Therefore, these disciplines seem most representative for researching saturation and mediatization in a statistically average environment.

The Spectrum and the Degree of Processual Saturation

In line with the adopted definition of mediated process,[16] the research aims to investigate which activities (consisting of sub-activities) saturate physical activities of the respondents. Based on that, a spectrum of mediated processes was specified and different variants of the degree of processual saturation were established.

The Spectrum

The survey showed that during physical activities, four main types of mediated processes occur:

- receiving and sending-receiving processes (receiving: listening to music, listening to the radio, watching TV, watching films, surfing the Internet; sending-receiving: making telephone calls),
- self-tracking: monitoring and analytical processes (analysis of data on one's own activity in real time),
- recording processes (photographing, filming), and
- interactive activating processes (playing video games).

It is also possible to single out a category of processes that make physical activity more attractive, which comprises of a mix of the above categories (e.g., using a drone, which can be used for recording and activating).

It is worth noting that sample data clearly shows there are no pure sending processes: e.g., sending SMS, MMS, publishing posts in social media etc. during the workout. It can be justified by the highly engaging character of such processes and the necessity to concentrate mainly on them, which makes it impossible to complete some of the physical activities. The survey showed, however, that communication related to physical activity takes place mainly after the activity.[17]

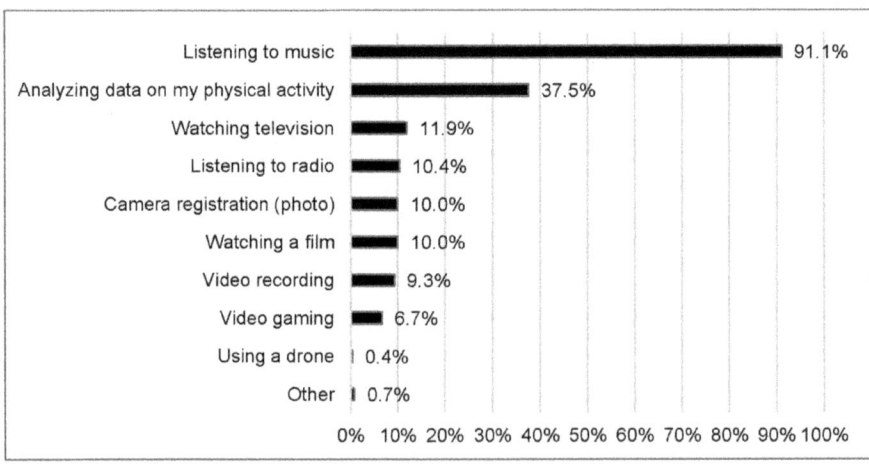

Figure 2.3.   This graph shows the saturation of physical activities with processes in the surveyed group. (N=269).

Source: Survey data. The percentage in the graph exceeds 100 since the participants could choose more than one response.

Listening to music is an accompanying activity in which a prevailing percentage (91%) of physically active participants engage. It is important to note that listening to music can be done with the use of many different devices (radio, television, music player); it can have a personalized character (one's own device, headphones) or not (music from speakers e.g., in a public place like a gym). In terms of its shareable nature, none of the aforementioned activities can equal to music while a much lower number of participants analyze their physical activity (37.5%). Again, it is worth noting that the analysis of one's own physical activity can have a different character, determined, yet not exclusively, by the use of media technologies (e.g., making traditional handwritten notes). Other, less popular activities included watching television (11.9%), listening to the radio (10.4%), and watching films (10%). Although, theoretically, in all three cases one can attempt to obtain instructions for training in real time through these media (e.g., an instructional film with a set of exercises), they are generally media that only accompany physical activity.

Quite notably, the number of recipients who watch television or films is higher compared to those who declare using these media. That discrepancy can partly derive from receiving a different number of responses to the question about accompanying activities as compared with the question about technologies used (269 versus 261). It might also suggest that the respondents are more aware of engaging in those activities than the fact of using particular devices to complete them.

Ten percent of respondents declare that they record their activity via photos and 9.3 percent declare that they film them. Playing video games, using a drone, and other (telephone conversations, surfing the Internet) can be classified as marginal activities.

Variants of the Degree of Processual Saturation

In order to specify the degree of processual saturation in the surveyed sample, the following variants of measuring saturation were proposed:

- the degree of individual processual saturation (IPS): the number of mediatized processes performed by a person divided by the number of mediatized processes which occur in the surveyed sample multiplied by 100 percent,

IPS = processes performed by a person ÷ number of mediatized processes · 100 percent

- the degree of processual saturation in the surveyed sample (PSS): the average number of mediatized processes in the surveyed sample divided by the number of mediatized processes which occur in the surveyed sample multiplied by 100 percent,

PSS = average number of mediatized processes ÷ number of mediatized processes · 100 percent

- the degree of processual saturation of a particular form of physical activity in the surveyed sample (PSPF): the average number of mediatized processes performed by respondents divided by the number of mediatized processes implemented by the respondents who engage in particular forms of physical activity in the surveyed sample multiplied by 100 percent.

PSPF = average number of mediatized processes ÷ number of mediatized processes in particular forms of physical activity · 100 percent

The possibilities to utilize the above calculations are parallel to the calculations of the degree of technological saturation with one difference: they assess the ability to perform a few processes simultaneously. While a number of the mediated processes can mean multitasking, part of the processes take place in the background of the physical activity and other processes are present only before the physical activity or after its completion. The calculations allow for comparing maximums, minimums, and average numbers within a sample and between various forms of physical activity while the results indicate the degree of processual complexity of physical activity.

The Results of Calculations

Table 2.2.   Variants of degree of processual saturation

The degree of individual processual saturation (IPS)	The degree of processual saturation of the surveyed sample (PSS)	Relative degree of processual saturation of a particular form of physical activity in the surveyed sample (PSFS)
IPS minimum: 1 ÷ 22 · 100% = 4.545% IPS maximum: 20 ÷ 22 · 100% = 90.90% (the result proceding the maximum: 12 ÷ 22 · 100% = 54.54%)	PSS: 3.82 ÷ 22 · 100% = 17.364%	PSFS running: 4.05 ÷ 22 · 100% = 18.409% PSFS gym: 3.8 ÷ 22 · 100% = 17.27%

Source: Own calculations based on survey data.

The calculations show that the spread between the maximum and the minimum IPS is very wide (4.545 percent and 90.90 percent), where IPS maximum may be treated as an aberration (arising from errors in filling out the question-naire). However, assuming the next highest number (54.54%) as correct, the spread still remains very wide. It indicates diverse models of doing physical activity, from hardly saturated processually to intensely saturated. PSS is 17.364 percent, which is a low number, but it refers to four mediated processes realized during physical activity. Similarly to technological saturation, the most popular forms of activity are characterized by PSFS similar to PSS.

By connecting the results obtained for both technological and processual saturation, it is evident that the relatively small degree of available technologies does not mean that the degree of mediated processes is equally low. It is dependent, among other factors, the multifunctionality of devices, but can also arise from the functional fit of media technologies to that form of human activity and a particular processual compatibility which is generated between physical activity and the use of technology. The mechanisms which favor that state require deeper analysis by qualitative research.

Media Saturation of Physical Activity—Qualitative Aspects

In order to specify the aspects of saturation, we have to indicate the characteristics of technologies and saturating processes. Positioned at the core of mutual relationships with the activities done by the respondents, they determine mediatization; in other words, they play a role in the mutual transformation of physical activity and media activity.

Technological Saturation

The quality of technological saturation can be seen as the structural quality of a technology reflected in the specification of its properties, including build, functionality, design, affordances, and other qualities that decide whether a technology is used and whether it plays a particular role in physical activity. In a survey method, that quality can be specified only in a very general sense. To examine it, the particular functions of technologies were examined in the population sample preceded by the evaluation of the importance of the media technologies. The obtained results were used for further qualitative research aimed at providing a more detailed insights into the process of saturation development and mediatization emergence.

The Importance of Particular Technologies

First, the rank of particular technologies in the surveyed sample was established to assess their importance during physical activities.

The highest rank (rank 1) was most often given to music players (44.8%) and smartphones (38.2%) followed by Endomondo application (4.1%). The second rank was most often awarded to smartphones (29.6%) and music players (28%), while the third place was given once more to Endomondo (8.8%), followed by watch tracker (3.8%). In the case of rank 3, the dispersion of responses was much higher. Mostly reported was Endomondo application (16.4%), cameras in smartphones (13.5%), and smartphones (10.4%). However, a significant percentage of surveyed respondents (4.5–6%) reported Internet radio, other mobile applications, video cameras in smartphones, and other cameras.

Three media technologies have a clearly dominating character in terms of their importance for the users: smartphone, music player, and Endomondo application, and they are most often given the first or the second rank by the users. One of the three ranked technologies shown on the third position was a camera in a smartphone.

Following the outcomes the obtained and analyzed results, the technologies were ordered according to the frequency in which they were given the first, the second, and the third rank. The number of indications in the study of the first, most important place has been multiplied by three; second place through two, so as to show which technologies are the most important for users. This resulted in a uniform hierarchization of technological solutions used in practice by individuals who regularly take up physical activity.

The first position was awarded to music player (413 points) while the second was given to smartphone (380 points). They were followed by significantly lower-ranked Endomondo application (81 points) and a camera in smartphones (40 points). Trackers (in watches) were listed often in the fifth position while the sixth was taken by Internet radio, followed by video cameras in smartphones.

While five of those technologies are regarded as leading are digital, mobile, and personalized, three of them show high technological and content convergence (smartphone, watch-tracker, Endomondo) and two are specifically dedicated to physical activity (Endomondo).

The functions of the technologies ranked as most important were examined in the next parts of the research. From the perspective of the hierarchy of importance of media technologies shaped in such manner, it was necessary to establish the properties of the technologies which decide about their importance in physical activity and its mediatization.

Functions of Technologies

In the survey, the respondents were asked what technology functions are most important for them during physical activity. Over three-quarters of the respondents observed the (1) motivating function of the technologies they used; on average one-third appreciate that they are useful in (2) analyzing and (3) archiving physical activity data, and one-quarter see that they are useful in (4) creating a training plan and (5) monitoring physical activity data during its progress (almost one-quarter of respondents).

From the perspective of five of those functions, and based on the researched sample, it can be stated that media technologies saturate physical activity due to the functions that cater to increasing its effectiveness, motivating for physical activity and operating data pertaining to physical activity (from archiving, through following results and modifying activity in real time, to analyzing data and training planning). These functions play a greater role than functions of social character, such as competitiveness, publishing, discussing, or keeping in touch.

Technology is more powerful in terms of effectiveness rather than in terms of making physical activity social, communicating about it, making it spectacular, or giving it other sense (e.g., charitable purposes). Multitasking, seen as using technology to increase the ability to perform several tasks simultaneously, also seems to be marginal. Physical activity, although saturated by media, generally remains a largely isolated activity and, as it appears from the indicated functions, it is deliberate and effectiveness-oriented.

However, upon closer investigation of the results of the most important functions of the technologies used during physical activity across different age groups, some differences can be observed. More participants aged between 20 and 24 years use technologies to increase the effectiveness of their training by creating training plans, monitoring and analyzing data during a training session, and archiving it to evaluate their progress than those from the age group of 15–19. Younger people use technologies more often to maintain social relationships during physical activity and to be able to engage in other, sports-unrelated activities during training. For them, technology has a more hybrid character as it combines effectiveness-related functions with social functions and multitasking. It might be said that the older respondents are, the more important the sport effects and results become.

Mediatization through Technological Saturation

The results of the research show that the influence of used media technologies is not radical[18] as it does not inflict changes on the practiced sport discipline. It is worth noting, however, that a small percentage of the respondents (5.5%) declared they switched to a different sport discipline under the influence of the technology they used.

Researching the relationship between the technology used and a radical change, for example changing the form of physical activity, did not indicate any particularly dominating technology. Yet, individuals who altered the form of exercise in which they engaged, or switched to a different physical activity altogether, indicated the change was triggered by the use of smartphones (nine people), mobile application Endomondo (four people), mobile application Nike+ (three people), mobile application Google Fit (three people), mobile application Runtastic (one person), movement sensor (one person), Kinect type video games (one person), drone (one person), a camera in a smartphone (two people), and a video camera in a smartphone (one person).

The influence of technologies saturating physical activity turned out to be less radical and resulted in impacting the frequency and intensity of physical activity. More than every third respondent declared that the media technology they used influenced the frequency of their physical activity, with the majority (32 percent of the total of physically active respondents) claiming that the frequency has increased while only 3.8 percent indicated a decrease. It must be emphasized that, among the remaining respondents, as many as 17.4 percent were not able to evaluate that influence. This means that overall, 46 percent of the respondents had no opinion on the influence of technology on the frequency of training sessions.

Participants who declared an increase in physical activity frequency most often used music players and smartphones (over 71%), Endomondo (40.2%), Nike+ (11.5%), a smartphone camera, and a GoPro camera (8%), while decreased frequency of physical activity was declared by those who most often used smartphones (60%), Endomondo (40%), and music players (40%).

Increasing and decreasing the frequency of physical activity seems to correlate with a similar set of media technologies that are used. The main listed three are: smartphone, music player, and Endomondo. The disputable meaning of the potential influence of technologies pertains to evaluating the quality of physical activity. Decreasing frequency of physical activity could mean that the training sessions are more effective and there is no need to do them as often as before technology became involved. It could also mean, however, that due to the use of technologies, the recipient achieved a satisfactory level of outcomes that subsequently resulted in lower frequency.

On the other hand, increased frequency does not necessarily translate into lowered effectiveness of training sessions and the need to schedule them more often. Playing music and engaging in other activities with the use of a smartphone or particular mobile applications may also enhance the pleasure and satisfaction users derive from sport activities and subsequently lead to increased training frequency regardless of the results.[19]

Independent of possible causes, quantitative change of physical activity accompanies high saturation with particular media technologies in the researched sample.

A similar dependency pertains to the intensity of physical activity. However, changes of frequency in training sessions were observed by one-third of physically active respondents, while half of them declared changes in training intensity. Over 45 percent of participants took up more intense physical activity as a result of media technologies use, whereas 2.3 percent declared lowered intensity. Finally, one-third of the total of physically active respondents stated that media technologies influenced the intensity of their training.

All in all, the usage of technology in physical activity increases its volume rather than decreases it, and its enhanced intensification varies across different forms of physical activity. A similar trend can be observed in the relationship between growing frequency or intensity and used technology.

It is worth noting that the attitude toward physical activity changes as well. Over 58 percent of the respondents who take up regular activity declared that using the media technology had a positive impact on their attitude to physical activity, with almost 17 percent declaring that difference in a definite manner, compared to only a little above 15 percent of respondents stating the opposite (almost 5 percent of them said "definitely no").

The comparison of responses to the above question (influence on improving your attitude toward physical activity) with particular technologies, regarded by the respondents as most important, did not give immediately obvious results.

Of respondents, 65.7 percent regarded music player as the most important media technology during physical activity and declared that their attitude to physical activity changed to more positive (including definite answers of 17.2 percent), with 47.6 percent smartphone users (including definite answers of 17.1 percent) seconding that view.

In the context of the second most important technology, the percentage of respondents unsure about the impact on their attitude was definitely larger (the response "neither yes," "neither no," was given by 35.3 percent of respondents). The lack of such influence was stated by 17.1 percent of respondents in relation to music players and 33.3 percent to smartphones. It would not be folly, therefore, to conclude that dominating technologies, with music players in particular, play a significant role in shaping up positive attitude in taking up physical activity.[20]

It is noteworthy that all respondents using mainly a smartphone camera noticed that the impact these technologies made on their more positive attitude toward physical activity. This can be influenced by the visualization function, which allows for the documentation of training sessions and their advancement, illustrating what progress has been made; and sometimes also a socializing and promotional function (in the case the material is published online), that fosters motivation for further effort.

Among the respondents who ranked smartphone camera as most important, one-third did not see the positive influence of that media technology on their attitude to physical activity and similar response was offered for those using Endomondo. It might be that their attitude toward physical activity is so firmly grounded, that the possibility of visualization, archiving or data analysis does not affect their stance.

In order to specify tangible implications of using key media technologies noticed by the respondents (i.e., the technologies indicated as the most important ones), the survey contained questions about the relationship between technology use and the improvement of their 1) physical condition/sport results, 2) health, and 3) appearance.

Forty-two percent of respondents stated that the media technologies they used contributed to the improvement of their physical condition and led to tangible results while 24.9 percent gave negative answers. It is worth noting that a similar percentage of respondents thought that the intensity of their workouts increased due to media technologies use (45.1%) and that their physical condition/sport results improved as well (42%).

The opinions about positive influence of the technologies used on the physical condition/sport results was most often expressed by people who use a watch tracker and a Go Pro camera. However, it has to be noted that relatively few respondents use these technologies. This could be due to their relatively high cost as they offer better visualization, archiving and analytical tools, and therefore those who use them may intend to professionalize their physical activity. Dominating technologies, i.e., music players, smartphones and Endomondo were regarded as fostering improving physical condition by 48 percent, 30.8 percent, and 44.4 percent, respectively.

When evaluating the influence of media technologies on improving health, positive responses were more frequent; however, the recognition of their advantages seemed much smaller (37.2 percent positive answers and 27.5 percent negative answers).

Most often, positive influence on health condition was noticed by people using smartwatches. A significant percentage of positive opinions was expressed also by people using Endomondo, music players, smartphones, and smartphone cameras; however, the percentage of positive opinions about those technologies is leveled by a similar percentage of negative opinions.

A very similar distribution of answers about the influence of the most important technology on health condition, was obtained in regards to the influence on appearance; equivocal answers dominated with positive answers ("definitely yes" and "rather yes") scoring 10 percent higher than the negative answers ("definitely not" or "rather not").

Concluding the answers about the influence of media technologies used during physical activity on physical condition, health, and appearance it has to be stated that the role of media technologies registered by the users is their effectiveness. On the one hand, respondents perceive the relationship between the influence on physical condition and results, but on the other hand, the respondents are not convinced that they influence physical condition and achieved results or they think that it is secondary role and they cannot specify it expressly.

The impact on these three areas (physical condition, health, appearance) is noticed in a similar degree as in the case of a music player (48%, 44%, 43% respectively) and smartphones (30,8%, 30,5%, 34,1% respectively). On the other hand, Endomondo, which is considered by some as significant in improving condition and health (44.4% and 44% respectively), is not considered as playing a part in improving appearance (22.2%). On the contrary: even more people indicate that there is no impact of this technology on physical condition, health, and appearance (44.5%, 44.5%, 44.4%, respectively).

There is a clear split in the observed impact of a smartphone video camera, which in the opinion of the researched people improves physical condition (66.6%) and appearance (66.6%), but not health (0%). Similarly perceived, although with a larger percentage of responses, is a GoPro camera (physical condition: 75 percent, appearance: 50 percent, health: 25 percent). The recording function of those monitoring and visualization technologies is, in some cases, related to growing importance of the aestheticizing of physical activity, which seems understandable, given the indicated technologies may serve as a means of documenting and presenting of the changes in the respondents' appearance.

Another notable fact is that unlike using a music player, listening to the radio cumulatively plays a role in fostering the improvement of the particular areas, i.e., condition, health, and appearance of physically active people. Although listening to the radio and listening to music are accompanying activities (they neither play a monitoring, documenting, or analytical role, nor foster an additional communicating activity), their perception differs significantly. The respondents indicate that music itself has a more profound impact on their physical activities. This might be due to the ability to choose one's playlist, and to listen to music only (as opposite to the hybrid word-music broadcast of a traditional radio program).[21]

Concluding the observations made so far, which pertain to the qualitative aspects of technological saturation, the analyzed surveys demonstrate the main directions of mediatization changes deriving from the interrelationship between media technologies and physical activity. The course usually flows from media technologies to physical activity and not the other way round. A peculiar technological "grammar" orientates physical activity to be more productive and makes it more effective. It is mainly shaped by the functions of technologies, but the extent of the role other characteristics of technologies (design, affordance, etc.) play in that transformation requires further defining.

Processual Saturation

Researching qualitative aspects of processual saturation, in other words grasping the specifics of mediated processes, is possible mainly by qualitative research methods. Defined antecedently by quantitative research results, those methods were carried out among members of particular sport-media worlds.[22] The preceding survey enabled the capturing of the mediated processes' specifics that accompany physical activity; the processes understood as communication about the respondent's physical activity and sport. In that context, it needs to be highlighted that most respondents indicated that they communicate about their physical activity after its completion (post factum) and not during its progress. Also, there were only a few respondents who declared the need to share their results with others (only 12 percent of respondents), the need to keep in touch during workout (8.9%), or to discuss their results (4.6%). When asked to indicate the technologies used to create and publish content referring to their physical activity, participants responded in various ways, as illustrated in Figure 2.4.

The results clearly demonstrate that the content pertaining to the respondents' own physical activity is most often published on Facebook (over 86%), followed by Snapchat (57.1%) and Instagram (53.5%), with one-third of participants using a smartphone camera for that purpose. However, this is where a significant contradiction has been observed, as only 12.6 percent of the respondents declared using a smartphone camera during physical activity. It is possible that, again, the discrepancy derives from lack of awareness of using a technology; in this case using a camera during physical activity. Publishing

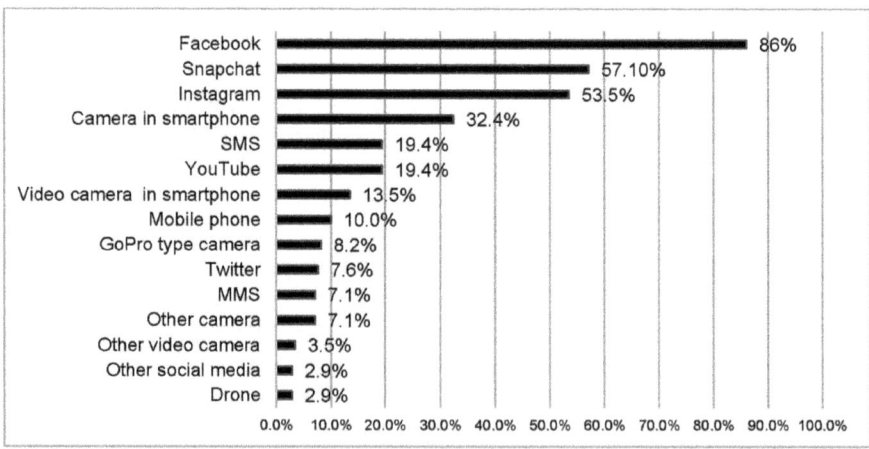

Figure 2.4.   Technologies used to create and publish texts, pictures, videos, and other content referring to respondents' own physical activity (N=170). The percentage in the graph exceeds 100 since the participants could choose more than one response.
Source: Survey data.

photos of the respondents' own activity (even if the photos are taken during the workout) are not treated as an element of that activity but as an independent task. It is also possible that photos are more often taken after the completion of or before the physical activity, but not during its course and for that reason those activities are isolated in the respondents' consciousness. The fact that the photos are published mainly post factum only supports that statement further.

The main three social media are picture-based, static, or moving (Instagram, Snapchat) or multimedia-oriented (Facebook) and thus communication about one's own activity is predominantly visual. Moreover, it takes place in the one-to-many model,[23] which contributes to reaching a potentially wide group of recipients.

Unsurprisingly, the three most important publishing technologies are social media and their choice differentiates across different age groups. Individuals aged between 20 and 24 years predominantly use Facebook (90%) and YouTube (22%) more often that people from the 15–19 age group (79% and 14%, respectively). On the other hand, participants from the younger group more often use Snapchat (80 percent versus 46 percent in the 20–24 group), Instagram (64 percent vs. 48 percent) and SMSs (27 percent vs. 17 percent). It shows that the younger the participants, the more elusive the technologies they use tend to be.

Mediated communication and physical activity converge to a limited degree as a separation of usage of media technologies in exercises and communication about physical activity can be observed, particularly in relation to more specialized technologies. The respondents who indicated specialized mobile applications or trackers as their most important media technologies used in physical activity communicate about their physical feats through media technologies only to a scant extent, which is surprising, particularly in terms of the affordance of automatic and intuitive relationship of services like Endomondo with e.g., Facebook, which offer incentives for fluid and immediate posting of results across several platforms simultaneously. In the researched cohort that does not happen: the possible incentives do not seem to have any effect.

By locating physical activity in the context of sport interests at large,[24] the ways media technologies are used to create and publish content were identified, with 64 percent of respondents disseminating sport-themed texts, photos, and videos.

In the analysis of technologies used to publish content about the respondents' own activity and other people's activity, social media dominate, leading with visual media (Snapchat, Instagram, YouTube) and most hybrid medium—Facebook. It is worth noting that Facebook is much more often used to publish content related to one's own activity whereas content about physical activity of others dominates on Twitter.

Content related only to physical activity of oneself is most often publicized with the use of Snapchat and Facebook (more than half of the respondents), followed by Instagram (48.2%) and YouTube (24.9%), with 44 percent of the respondents using a smartphone camera to create and publish posts.

In terms of creating and publishing sports related content of others, two age populations were also compared and several distinctions have been observed. Participants between 20 and 24 years old use a smartphone camera or a video camera as well as a GoPro camera more often than participants from the group aged between 15 and 19 years. On the other hand, the latter group uses Snapchat, Twitter, Facebook, and SMSs more often than individuals from the older group. This confirms the tendency of younger people to favor channels of more ephemeral character and a strictly social nature as opposed to the documenting and independent character of the recording tools (video cameras and cameras) preferred by participants from the older group.

Mediatization Through Processual Saturation

As aforementioned, the research based on questionnaires was mainly focused on transforming physical activity as a result of using media technologies. The opposite process, referring to the impact of physical activity on changes in media and communication, is rather secondary and indirect as demonstrated in the following section.

Based on the questionnaires results, it can be stated that mediatization of physical activity occurs directly and indirectly and its specifics depend on media saturation. While direct mediatization takes place through technological saturation, indirect mediatization occurs due to processual saturation. In the former case, the transformation of physical activity is facilitated by the presence and usage of a particular technology, resulting in physical activity extending beyond traditional body movement with the use of its muscles.[25] It becomes a body movement intertwined with the media technology in the material and structural sense. In other words, classic body movement turns into a directed, modeled activity, transformed by technology, which mediates particular stages within that process. In the former case, however, mediatization has a direct character because using media technology facilitates mediation of the given processes (sequence of activities and actions) and through that mediation their transformation takes place. The use of technology results in, for example, a change of schedule and training plan (e.g., frequency of physical activity) and the course of physical activity (e.g., intensity of physical activity).

In terms of indirect mediatization, the transformation of physical activity is based on mediated communication. One of the mediated processes taking place during physical activity comprises of communication about its results, including registering and analyzing data, as well as improving one's attractiveness. Physical activity is often accompanied, and even more often preceded or completed by, communication about it. Its format is diverse (text based, pictorial, video-based, multimedia-based) and disseminated with the use of different information flow models (one-to-one, one-to-many, many-to-many, hybrid). As a result, communication about physical activity changes respondents' perception of it, the perception of particular disciplines (e.g., their rules), their identity and the culture they generate, including trends, patterns, and norms. In that sense, physical activity is mediatized with media-generated structure providing the basis of this activity and its transformation.

This media structure is fluxional and dynamic due to the material presence of changeable and diverse technologies. Physical activity, including numerous particular sport disciplines, as well as the communicated and constructed sport-media worlds, are inhomogeneous. In many cases, they are highly individualized, although with distinctive variations; they can be mass, egalitarian, but also niche or elitist.

While the aforementioned aspects focused on qualitative, processual properties of saturation of physical activity facilitating direct and indirect mediatization, the following chapter discusses subsequent, qualitative surveys that examine in detail particular factors conditioning that process.

NOTES

1. The forms of movement under investigation were selected on the basis of data from national statistical surveys, mainly: *Aktywność Fizyczna Polaków* BS/129/2013. http://www.cbos.pl/SPISKOM.POL/2013/K_129_13.PDF (retrieved online).

2. The research was carried out between 15 May 2016 and 15 July 2016.

3. The results of the tests, which constituted the basis for constructing the test sample, are included in Appendix 1.

4. For detailed results, please refer to Appendix 1.

5. Gumpert, Gary and Cathcart, Robert, "Media Grammars, Generations, and Media Gaps," *Critical Studies in Media Communication* 2.1 (1985): 23–35. Göran Bolin, "The Rhythm of Ages: Analyzing Mediatization Through the Lens of Generations Across Cultures," *International Journal of Communication* (10) (2016): 5254–55.

6. However, there are also surveys which include respondents as young as 7 years old, e.g., Deloitte Digital, "Raport Strategiczny. Internet 2015/2016," (retrieved online).

7. In Poland, research is carried out mainly on a group of adults (from 18 years of age) since they do not require informed consent by parents or guardians.

8. Detailed justification of the choice of population and the survey sample, including the calculations of its representativeness are included in Appendixes 1 and 2.

9. The details and calculations of the population sample are to be found in Appendix 2.

10. More at Joshua Meyrowitz, *No Sense of Place: The Impact of Electronic Media on Social Behavior* (New York: Oxford University Press, 1986), 69.

11. Herbert Kubicek, "Das Internet auf dem Weg zum Massenmedium? Ein Versuch, Lehren aus der Geschichte alter und anderer neuer Medien zu ziehen," in "Modell Internet? Entwicklungsperspektiven neuer Kommunikationsnetze," ed. Raymund Werle and Christa Lang (Frankfurt a.M., New York: Campus Verlag, 1997) in Andreas Hepp, *Cultures of Mediatization* (Cambridge, MA: Polity Press, 2013), 4.

12. John Rooksby et al., *"Personal Tracking as Lives Informatics,"* in *Proceedings of the 32nd Annual ACM Conference on Human Factors in Computing Systems* (Toronto: ACM, 2014): 1165–66.

13. And potentially drawing comparisons between samples, especially in time periods, and further, selecting the particular respondents or their equivalents for qualitative survey.

14. Subsequently, calculating the average numbers obtained from a sample enables specifying the degree of technological saturation (TSS), which may be used to draw comparisons between samples (different samples per age, place of residence, etc.), in particular considering time periods to observe the quantitative changes over time.

15. TSFS enables considering the survey results in comparative analyses between samples, e.g., over an extended period of time as well.

16. A sequence of mediated activities and/or actions stretched out in time which cause changes.

17. More in chapter 3 and chapter 4.

18. Radical influence should be understood as the essential and deep change in an activity; in the case of physical activity it could mean abandoning it or changing the form of physical activity. Since the research was carried out among physically active people, the number of individuals who completely abandon physical activity due to the media technologies they used could not be estimated.

19. Those traits were analysed in the qualitative survey in the next research stage. See chapter 4.

20. It is an indication to further examine the causes of that influence those technologies make. See chapter 3.

21. The significance of music however, requires further research to establish the sources of its significance for mediatization of physical activity.

22. Chapters 6 and 7.

23. Merrill Morris and Christine Ogan, "The Internet as Mass Medium," *Journal of Computer-Mediated Communication*, 1 (4) (1996), https://doi.org/10.1111/j.1083-6101.1996.tb00174.x.

24. Not only taking into consideration interests in sport manifested in activity (e.g., taking up one's own physical activity) but also in a passive manner (e.g., observing other people's activity).

25. "Physical activity is defined as any bodily movement produced by skeletal muscles that requires energy expenditure," WHO, "Physical Activity" (retrieved online).

Chapter Three

Qualitative Specification of Physical Activity Media Saturation

Dominating Forms of Physical Activity and Popular Technologies

The quantitative survey on the media saturation of physical activity carried out among young individuals revealed dominating and niche media-sports worlds. Running and exercising at the gym proved to be most popular activities, while media technologies dominating physical activity comprised of smartphones, music players, and sport self-trackers (mainly Endomondo). The first stage of qualitative research was thus directed at exploring the media-sports worlds that emerge relatively often on the intersection of the aforementioned activities and technologies.

The aim of the research was to identify the characteristics of technological and processual saturation in the area dominating the surveyed cohort. Based on the survey data, first the specifics of physical and technological activity of gym users and runners were explored by comparison to the antecedently obtained data. The comparisons are considered to be indicative due to the limited sample size comprising of the respondents declaring their most important activities (gym exercises: seventy-six vs. running: forty). The sample value is encompassed by its supportive function in setting out the direction of qualitative research (with an in-depth, semi-structured interviews) and subsequently allowing for the characteristics of technological and processual saturation to be established.

It was revealed that 19 percent of gym users do not take up any other form of physical activity, while the majority of the sample participants widen the scope of the sports they engage with running, riding a bicycle, or playing football identified as most popular. On the other hand, among runners only 3 percent of people do not engage in any other sports. Most runners often ride a bicycle, go to the gym, or play football.

Runners often do other exercise, and people who exercise often run and, subsequently, the worlds of runners and gym users often overlap. Moreover, other forms of physical activity than running and gym exercises enrich those worlds. For that reason, those worlds have been categorized as multidisciplinary.

The comparison of ranks ascribed to the most important media technologies of the gym goers and runners is similar to the overall results from the entire survey cohort. For both the gym goers and runners, the three most important technologies used during physical activity are smartphones, music players, and the Endomondo application. The difference between those two activities pertains to the first technology: gym goers favor smartphones while runners use mainly music players.

The obtained results allowed for the separation of sport-media worlds of runners and gym goers, with both groups listening to music on a music player or a smartphone while engaged in a physical activity. The domination of those two sports technologies played a deciding role in separating a field that allows for a deepened analysis of most popular practices among young people. At the same time, it allowed for the exploration of the qualitative aspects of media saturation in the most popular sport-media world.

In the context of the aforementioned survey results, individual in-depth semi-structured interviews were carried out[1] with the respondents displaying the following characteristics:

- comparative demographics to the preceding surveys: 15–24 years old (divided into two age groups: 15–19 and 20–24) residents of a large urban agglomeration,[2]
- declared frequency and intensity of physical activity similar to the sample in the preceding surveys: gym exercises and running at least once a week for at least sixty minutes a week,
- a habit of listening to music on a music player or a smartphone during physical activity.

After completing the interview, the respondents were asked to take photos of the equipment they use during running or exercising at the gym next time they train, resulting in 63 percent of respondents sending their photos for analysis.

The cohort comprised of nineteen respondents,[3] including: eight men and eleven women; nine of them from the younger age group (up to 19 years old) and ten people from a group aged between 19 and 24 years. Twelve people declared that running is their main form of physical activity versus nine people favoring gym sessions. The respondents represented various configurations of the sports in which they engaged:

- only running (three participants),
- only gym exercises (four participants),
- running and gym exercises (two participants),

- running, exercising at the gym and other sport or sports (six participants),
- running and other sport or sports (three participants),
- gym exercises and other sport or sports (one participants).

Participants who took part in the interviews represented diverse sport interests (maximum number of activities was five, with two on average), but some were focused on one type of physical activity. The cohort differentiated in terms of additional activities taken up by respondents which included: fitness, exercising at home, boxing, hurdles, bicycling, football, volleyball, basketball, skiing, and diving.

The majority of respondents (seventeen out of nineteen) use their smartphones to listen to music during their physical activity. While most of them (eleven out of nineteen) used Endomondo, two favored other, yet similar applications (Nike Plus, Runtastic). Only two individuals did not indicate using other media technologies than a personal music player and Endomondo. Most of them (seventeen out of nineteen) used several other media technologies (from twp to eight) with the complete spectrum of the technologies used in the research cohort reaching eighteen.

Concluding, the respondents comprised of a diverse group: multidisciplinary in terms of sport activities and relatively interdisciplinary in terms of the media technologies they used.

The media-sports worlds of gym goers and runners, who use music player type of technologies during physical activity, initially revealed in the surveys and further explored during the interviews, made it possible to specify the quality of media saturation, with the distinction between technological saturation and processual saturation made.

TECHNOLOGICAL SATURATION

As aforementioned, technological saturation (structural saturation) is understood as the way in which technology saturates its immediate environment in practice due to its properties, with the focus on functionalities, design, and affordances.[4]

Smartphonization of Physical Activity

The research demonstrated that, despite the wide spectrum of technologies used in physical activity, technologies favored by runners and gym goers were mainly multifunctional, universal, and used during other activities and circumstances, too; they comprised mainly smartphones. The interviewees valued the simplicity and user-friendly experience of their tools above the sophisticated features and higher specialization of the devices. In other words, they favored technologies that can be described as basic and popular. Some of them expressed a wish to widen the spectrum of the technologies they used, with a preference given to "trendy" gadgets such as smartwatch.

The basic characteristic of media technologies that is decisive for their practicality in physical activity is their handiness: participants favor devices that are small and easy to carry, e.g., in a pocket. Such properties make media technologies mobile, allowing for them to be placed near one's body and used in almost every situation, with this view explicitly expressed by one of the respondents:

> "You always have a phone with you, and putting on headphones and putting the phone in your pocket is not a problem" (male participant 5).

It is worth noting that across the entire cohort of respondents, the primary goal lies in minimalizing the number of devices. On the one hand, it stems from seeking maximum comfort as during any physical activity individuals lack suitable space to store their devices, they risk of damage of loss increases and they can become a burden during movement—a complaint particularly widespread among owners of larger smartphones. The respondents claim that "a lot of equipment gets in the way." Therefore, one multifunctional device is more effective than many individual gadgets that have to be used separately and secured, which, unsurprisingly, is perceived as highly inconvenient.

Moreover, smartphones are a memory relieving technology that reduces users' memory burden. For example, the users no longer have to remember about performing numerous tasks in preparation for their workout (charging the battery, plugging in the accessories, downloading special applications and content) or those related to storage and protection (e.g., from damage or theft) of special equipment to listen to music:

> "I always have a telephone on hand and when I go to the gym, I do not have to be afraid of forgetting it" (male participant 1).

Moreover, using a smartphone during exercise allows for engagement in other activities, such as answering phone calls, accessing data and downloading content ("it's my memory stick"). That device always accompanies the user and thus becomes indispensable and ever-present. It is therefore natural and obvious for users to always carry their smartphones. While other technologies can be viewed and treated as expendable, this does not apply to smartphones.

Apart from physical properties deriving from devices' construction and design, the relationships between these two elements and the resulting affordances appear to be equally important; above all, the encouragement to use smartphones in particular ways.

The convenience of downloading content online, including mostly music, is an incentive to use the device as a music player. Free mobile apps foster that with premium versions offering widened access to selected content (e.g., without ads) which often does not require having internet access. Also, paid applications enable high personalization of content, which seems to be of paramount importance in the context of physical activity, leading to this affordance being regarded as highly positive.

In addition, having built-in cameras and video cameras and integrating a smartphone with social network platforms, such as Facebook, Instagram, Snapchat brings users the affordance for documenting and (sometimes almost automatic) publishing content, especially across those platforms. Physical activity becomes monitored and visual data undergoes archiving, analysis, and exchange in the process of communication. However, the encouragement to record one's own physical activity and posting the outcomes is not always regarded as positive. While it is viewed as an important tool for self-improvement, motivation, and self-presentation, it is also seen as a distractor. Instead of exercising users constantly record their physical activity and often publicize the materials and even discuss them during exercise. This is regarded as very distracting and can evoke irritation in potential recipients of that content:

> "I don't support this style: 'Hi! I came to the gym and I'm taking a photo. . .Hi! I did three squats. . .Hello! I'm going to the mirror now . . . I finished my workout and I'm leaving. . ." (female participant 4).

Similarly, not all respondents were entirely positive about the possibility of constant internet connection deriving from smartphones' ownership and applicable subscription charges. Most were either positive or neutral about it, praising mainly the option of free application downloads, including mostly music with particular emphasis on the newest releases. However, the respondents also noticed that their activity is strongly dependent on internet access and its content and they expressed the need to use offline or even analogue technologies. One participant, for example, justified using an analogue stepper (step counting device), so that she "doesn't have to worry about the phone" and that she is "independent of the internet and all the frills of today's world."

Some respondents, despite carrying a smartphone with free, subscription-based apps designed for tasks data collection during their workouts, record them in traditional notebooks or copybooks. Interestingly, however, there were no negative comments regarding the need to connect to the Internet to use smartphone functionalities or applications and despite the cost incurred from having online access secured, none of the respondents mentioned it. The problem of its value is mainly linked to concerns over damage or theft, which is perceived as a real threat when using a smartphone during a work-out. Some people use a different phone (less valuable, older, or damaged), so to minimize that threat or they switch from a smartphone to a music player (mainly mp3 players). Only a few consider giving up some smartphone functionalities and using additional equipment, such as a smartwatch, but those are in minority.

What appears to be the biggest source of stress and frustration seems to derive from an unsatisfactory length of battery life. Less often users are vexed with insufficient amount of memory required to use the device during physical activity without restrictions and the possibility of being suddenly cut off from its functionality. Hence, some participants, despite the practical disadvantages, use several devices during their workout, including a smartphone for particular applications (mainly Endomondo) since the "app consumes a lot of power," and a separate player to listen to music.

The Importance of Accessories

A particular extension of smartphone new possibilities is provided by its accessories. In the researched cohort, the most important accessory were headphones used for listening to music; most often in the form of cable sets and rarely wireless. Headphones, an example of obvious technology that makes it almost "transparent," were most commonly used medium the respondents used while listening to music. It seems, therefore, natural for them to have headphones connected to their smartphones. Interestingly enough, when asked to photograph their entire equipment prior to and after a training session, they included the headphones, too, although not all respondents did that.

The informants usually use earphones, rarely traditional headphones,[5] which are a material and technological extension of a smartphone placed in the user's body. They are very small and placed close to the acoustic organ—inside the ear. They fit in tight, with some featuring an additional clip-on to fasten behind the ear so that they do not fall out during movement. They integrate with their owners, facilitating their acoustic isolation from the surroundings, which seems of paramount importance during physical activity. Earphones, therefore, are seen as the type of accessory that guarantees individual reception—"only for myself."

While in some situations headphones are necessary to listen to music, sometimes they merely allow for more comfort since users can hear better, and, most importantly, they can listen to the music they want to hear.[6] It is worth noting the non-acoustic meaning headphones bear. Some respondents declared that wearing their headphones was as important as the music itself since they got used to the feeling and thus the accessory became indispensable. In situations when they cannot listen to music during a workout (e.g., because their battery is depleted) they put their earphones on or leave them in their ears to continue on with their workout even though there is no sound coming out:

"I associate that feeling in my ears with listening to music and it helps me in some way" (male participant 1).

The above clearly demonstrates that media technologies are meaningful not due to their content only, but also due to their design or functions. The content (music, audiobooks, radio program) are the sole reason the technology is used at all, but playing a particular function in a user's physical activity arises from their plainly material properties, too. Headphones are a communication channel (to listen to music), but are also an acoustic, and sometimes even mental, isolator.

It is worth noting that the technology in the provided photographs was not featuring slipcovers, cases, bands, or armbands despite the respondents declaring their use. Also, any other accessories were not mentioned since they are treated as natural, and thus "transparent." Accessories, therefore, actually model physical activity to a significant extent. A smartphone armband strapped on before a run allows the users to glance at the screen at any given time, without interrupting the activity, making unnecessary movements, or without risking dropping the device.

This seemingly small change—the possibility to wear a device on one's body or gear, not necessarily carried in a pocket, but much more easily accessible, plays an important role in processual saturation of physical activity. A smartphone, along with an armband, shows affordances encouraging a particular action. The possibility of monitoring exercise with ease while engaging in other activities (answering phone calls, selecting a music piece, etc.) reinforces the eagerness to use a media technology during physical activity and widens the spectrum of technologies used (mostly mobile applications). As a result, and through integration with technologies used to communicate about that physical activity, it leads to even stronger mediatization. In particular, easy accessibility and convergence of technologies stimulate respondents to use sport trackers like Endomondo, which strongly models physical activity which can be illustrated by the following account:

"I've bought an arm-band and it's easy to turn my head and see the time and the number of kilometers. Especially when I'm in an intense workout, to beat a record, if I want to break my own 'record' time" (male participants 1).

Material properties of a medium, in other words its accessories, decide about the effectiveness of physical activity. The easy access to data (in this case requiring only a user's glance at the smartphone screen) decides about a drop or an increase of motivation in a given moment, and, later on, about the result, e.g., breaking a record. That, in turn, determines the feeling of satisfaction, which plays a deciding role in terms of the activity being continued or modified.

Interestingly enough, smartwatch users (complementing or substituting a smartphone in the described scope) have not reflected on the peculiar affordance embedded in that device. By imitating a traditional watch through its design and location on the wrist, a smartwatch encourages its user to look at its "face" whenever they need a piece of information. However, it does not result in users engaging with this device during their workouts. While they declared that a smartwatch can complement or substitute a smartphone, it is not used during a workout, but mostly afterward.

The respondents who did not mention using armbands or similar accessories also refrained from using sport self-trackers applications. However, when Endomondo was used via a smartphone placed in a pocket, engaging with the application had a different character during the run or a workout, yet played a similar role afterward, with the users checking their results, workout conditions, statistics, etc.

The Importance of a Playlist

In terms of technology saturation with smartphones, the key functionality appeared to be playing music. Equally important was the ability to easily download and store large music files on one multifunctional device and the convenience of updating the content by adding new items. In some cases, the possibility to download applications that offer various music genres, including premium versions that eliminate advertisements was of paramount importance. The respondents indicated the need for constant connection to the Internet to listen to music provided by smartphones, however they were appreciative of the possibility to create their own "music libraries" that eliminate the need for online access.

A key feature for respondents was a playlist, with the majority creating their own sets of music pieces on their phones and adapting the content to their individual needs. Smartphones feature such functionalities by default, but there is also a number of downloadable applications, such as Spotify or Tidal. In some cases, music is downloaded directly from YouTube. The users create their favorite playlists or use other people's playlists which, in turn, develops their own music interests. Since diversifying one's playlists is important to avoid boredom, respondents often search for new music pieces.

This is when suggestions made by applications can serve as a source of inspiration, resulting in enriching both the played content and the physical activity.

A smartphone featuring applications to create one's playlists allows for complete personalization of the music library—a strong need highlighted by many respondents. It seems, therefore, that creating a playlist becomes an important part of workout preparation. Hence, selecting particular music pieces is not accidental and is strictly tied to workout plans and other aspects surrounding physical activity.[7] Despite some respondents opting for music to be played at random, it is still selected from within the content of their own library. However, they might reach out to external media content providers, such as YouTube when boredom creeps in.

The Continuous Impact of Technologies Used to Listen to Music

In the researched group, smartphone is the dominating technology used for listening to music; that pertains to both runners and gym goers. The domination is stronger among the runners, which can derive from the fact that gyms are often featured with speakers, hence offering an alternative to one's own music by default. Gym goers, therefore, display a more liberal attitude toward playlists than runners. However, only the minority relies entirely on the music offer available at the gym and thus without demonstrating or fulfilling the aforementioned need to have a personalized playlist accompanying their workout. Nevertheless, all respondents listen to music during physical activity and they acknowledge its role in the modeling of physical activity.[8]

The continuous influence of technologies used for listening to music ranges from low impact in situations when music is treated as a dispensable addition, medium impact (when technology helps in activity), high impact (when it's a key supporting factor), and, finally, very high impact when technology conditions physical activity. Most notably, the complete lack of impact of technology or even the need for no technology does not take place as illustrated in Table 3.1.[9]

The analysis of the outlined continuum from its most extreme impact perspective shows that individuals, who condition their workouts on using audio technologies, engage in sport without music only "accidentally" or "when

Table 3.1.   Variants of the importance of media technologies in physical activity.

(It's not there or even it shouldn't be there)	*It could not exist*	*It helps or helps a lot*	*Absolute conditioning*
RESIGNATION OR NEGATION	AMBIVALENCE	REINFORCEMENT	CONDITIONING

Source: own elaboration.

the phone runs out of battery in the middle [of a workout] (. . .), never on purpose." The most extreme representation of this condition is illustrated by an even more orthodox stance on the matter: "Never. I always need to have music when I run."

> "When you're at a shooting range you could get by, but at the gym, or running without music, I don't know how you could do that. It's too quiet, empty, I feel uncomfortable and lost" (female participant 4).

Forgetting one's equipment or failing to charge it can lead to anger and frustration: "I try not to think about it because it annoys me that I was so absent-minded and forgot." Every physical activity is considered as generally of a lower quality if it is not accompanied by music. Participants who consider listening to music key or helpful can still do sports in silence, but the lack of its accompaniment is a cause for distress:

> "How did you feel then?"
> "Definitely bad. Running without music is weak. It's hard to workout, run or cook [sic!] without music . . ." (female participant 3).

> "It's happened that in the middle of a workout my battery died. I didn't get angry with the gym but I had the impression that exercising wasn't as good" (male participant 2).

Shortcomings of technologies can also cause disappointment with workouts deprived of music. For example, one respondent recounted an experience when new headphones, which had not been tested prior to a workout, turned out to be a bad fit. While it did not make the respondent finish the workout earlier, it made him dissatisfied with his training.

On the opposite spectrum are individuals who perceive audio technologies only as an insignificant addition, but they are a definite minority.[10] They state that music is neutral for them and the lack of a phone or earphones does not bother them. Due to the absence of technologies, the world will "not collapse" and they "don't care." This is even more evident in the case of gym goes, who resign from using personalized playlists with relative ease since music at the gym is provided.

Sport Self-trackers and Other Media Technologies

The second most important functionality of a smartphone in the context of physical activity is the ability to download and use mobile sport applications. They fulfill a variety of self-tracking features: monitoring, analyzing, coaching, often combined with social functions. Among the respondents, the most popular application of that type is Endomondo.

Saturation with sports trackers occurs in a two-fold manner: it derives from functionalities used in real time as well as from a wide scope of functionalities deployed either after a workout completion or during its preparation stage.

In the researched sample, Endomondo (and similar applications) is used mostly for monitoring concurrent results: the distance made, the speed, burned calories, and the pulse. These parameters are taken into consideration during physical activity and they shape its progress. One of the respondents saw it as "private coaching" since the application sent her alerts when her tempo was too slow, prompting her to accelerate to meet the target speed. That function, according to participants, is particularly important when aiming for a particular target during a workout, e.g., breaking their individual record. Therefore, controlling parameters is key for making decisions during a workout and the application delivers that automatically. It functions both as a long-term recording and a real-time data analysis device.

An application like that also gives users feedback on their progress. The application becomes a judge and a source of validation of the results achieved. Quite strikingly, none of the respondents questioned those analytical abilities or the subsequent results credibility. Such apps can prove that a workout has been effective, that progress has been made, as well as give meaning to the physical activity one does. They influence the feeling of satisfaction and encourage to continue training, given the ability to plan and use it rationally:

> "(. . .) running has even more sense when I put on Endomondo because I see my results and I can check many things" (female participant 3).

Some sport trackers also provide real-time tips as well as rewards, and while many respondents see it as nice-to-have, they are not perceived as significant functionalities. Quite surprisingly, most participants did not even reflect on the additional motivation those functionalities could potentially introduce to their workouts.

Among other media technologies used for running and gym training, the respondents made a distinction between those used in real time and those deployed before or after a workout. The first group comprised mainly of the following:

Monitoring and Analytical Technologies

- trackers: pedometers used to count steps; pulse meters a consisting of a chest strap and a specialized watch registering and analyzing pulse),
- smartwatches (multifunction devices),

- virtual reality trainers, e.g., devices that inform you about the distance, weight, counting body composition, calories burned,

Instructing Technologies

- applications dedicated to particular gym exercises (e.g., doing push-ups, squats, pull-ups),
- live streaming instruction (e.g., on YouTube), used during exercising at home,

Registering Technologies

- cameras and video cameras in smartphones,
- technologies enriching/diversifying physical activity: other applications, e.g., PokemonGo.

The group is complemented with technologies used in other sports, e.g., monitoring and analytical movement chips mounted on shoes, and applications enhancing the attractiveness of physical activity due to their social features or a charity-oriented focus.

The second group comprised of technologies used before or after a workout, such as instruction videos helping to prepare for weight training.[11]

In terms of functionalities, trackers (pedometer, pulse meter) are technologies that can be eliminated by using mobile smartphone applications. However, they can be used by individuals who intentionally choose devices beyond smartphones and other electronics.[12] Another technology that can substitute or supplement those is a smartwatch, most often integrated with applications installed on a smartphone. All in all, sport trackers structure physical activity, make it more systematic, effective, and increase the drive for doing it, e.g., using body composition tools conveys the message that "your workout has some sense."

It is worth emphasizing that broadcasting and instructive technologies (mainly videos on YouTube) turned out much less important than sport trackers. They can be used only in a place with the Internet access. They also require a bigger screen (a tablet, a laptop, a TV set) and a speaker, restricting their use to exercise at home or before a workout. The instructions, including guidance for the correctness of exercise, still remain a domain of another person—a coach or an instructor—whose expertise was recognized by some of the respondents. However, they comprise of a minority, which leads to the conclusion that results and data provided by technology are more valued than a direct interaction with a specialist. Moreover, they evaluate the quality of the effects independently (based on the data collected and photos or videos they took by themselves) or by getting social approval from friends.[13]

The last category includes technologies that enhance the attractiveness of physical activity. In the researched cohort, one respondent stood out as a user of the PokemonGo application. It is a mobile game featuring augmented reality with highly competitive elements directly linked to physical performance of players. The success is conditioned by the results of physical activity although the game is not dedicated to sports enthusiasts per se. However, it does motivate players to change their location, and hence it becomes an additional source of motivation to take up and continue physical activity. Also, the game features a peculiar registering affordance. The respondent, who used PokemonGo, used the video camera to record a Pokemon, i.e., a character from an augmented reality game. By recording the surrounding reality enhanced by the virtual elements while running, physical activity became highly hybridized and converged.

PROCESSUAL SATURATION

As aforementioned, processual saturation is seen as the way mediated processes occur in practice and their properties facilitate mediatization.

Listening to Music

Listening to music on one's own player during physical activity is a complex process, including both physical and mental dimension. This is predominantly a motivational process; it motivates individuals to begin physical activity, continue it, and increase its intensity.

Based on the answers of the respondents, the main flow of that process can be reconstructed. Preparing the player before the workout and putting earphones on initiates the process. It is a determining stage as in cases when the use of earphones is prevented by workout length,[14] other people's company,[15] or simply due to the lack of relevant equipment,[16] the respondents forgo listening to music and the following steps of the process do not take place.

The action of putting earphones on and the anticipation and certainty of the subsequent music flow serves as an activity trigger ("just the pure fact that I'll put on my earphones and will listen to something . . ."). Starting to listen to music (or even being aware that it will happen in a moment) is the first kind of motivation: motivation to start physical activity. For some respondents it arises from the pure pleasure of listening to music that accompanies the workout and, while most of them indicated their playlist were very diverse and they demonstrated no preference for any kind of genre or artist, [17] some named particular music genres they excluded. [18] Also, they experienced pleasure from listening to the same song repeatedly, and sometimes from searching for new, enticing tunes, and dedicating their run or exercise time to familiarize themselves with the newly sourced music.

Quite unanimously, respondents declared that music kept them busy, made time flow faster, eliminated the feeling of a potential time waste, and prevented boredom during exercise. Although in the minority, some respondents decidedly consider exercise without music (or other audio content such as the radio or audiobooks) a waste of time:

> "I can't imagine running without something playing, it would be a waste of time" (female participant 7).

Among the majority of respondents, the dominating motivational aspect of music lies within its power to boost their will to continue (or finish) the planned workout:

> "It is not about no motivation to work out, but about defeating, limiting or getting rid of the doubt that I can't make it" (male participant 2);

> "Energetic songs in a weird way give me strength for the next kilometers" (male participant 1);

> "If I want to quit, something is in that music that I still want to continue my workout" (female participant 4).

The respondents seem unable to explain why music plays such a big role in their workout and, on the whole, they do differentiate between the levels of importance of the musical and lyric aspect in songs.

In terms of lyrics, those "full of sense and meaning," "with a message," "thought-provoking," "wise lyrics that remind you of something important," and "with which I agree emotionally" bear some significance as they start a thought process that becomes integral with exercise, subsequently influencing its course and duration. Participants declared they were "sensitive to" words, lyrics "agitate to do more," and helped overcome their weaknesses.

The purely musical aspect, referring mainly to rhythm and tempo, and in particular in repetitive sequences with linear melody climaxes and falls, acts as a strong motivational trigger to intensify physical activity. The rhythm helps to achieve or extend its duration and stimulates to increase effort, overcome weaknesses, and achieve set targets. In other words, music helps develop physical abilities:

"When I'm running and I can't go anymore and there's that drop, I can squeeze more out of myself. (. . .) [When I listen to music] I try to have a longer workout, run one more loop etc." (male participant 4);

"Thanks to music I can get the rhythm, especially when I don't have motivation, when I've run a number of kilometers . . ." (female participant 5).

All in all, it seems that the levels of the impact the lyrics and music have on physical activity are hard to overestimate. There is no doubt that music and movement become integrated and influence one another; they are not isolated phenomena and they do not work unilaterally. For participants, the choice of music arises from a plan, the course, and the workout stage, but is also influenced by habits, mood, or the ordinary life experience of a particular day. Regardless of the music choices made, they impact physical activity to a great extent by influencing its duration, course, engagement levels, intensity, and the overall effectiveness. Two main functions play a decisive role in that context: music acting as an isolator and a modulator simultaneously.

Music has a high potential to become an isolator in two aspects: materially due to physical aspects of media technologies (earphones, the handiness of a player or smartphone) and, in nonmaterial form, due to the media content (music). A runner or a gym goer first isolate themselves from the surroundings, from other people, and from noise or from silence and this facilitates their solitude while exercising with music:

"I listen to music when I run, I turn myself off to other stimuli which may disrupt my workout" (male participant 5);

"When you have music you can separate yourself from anything" (male participant 3).

That isolation allows to focus in different ways. While it helps to concentrate on physical activity, it can directly and concurrently satisfy other aims; for example, it can calm one down or invigorate them. Music is chosen to fit a situation that often stems not only from the workout aims but from what an individual needs in a given moment. People who are upset want to calm down and those who feel sluggish want to liven up:

"[Music] stirs me up to exercise. (. . .) it gets my adrenaline flowing" (male participant 2);

"If I have nothing weighing on me or no problems during the day, or I know the next day is going to be light (. . .) I run slowly and I'm chilled. I put on calmer music (. . .) But when I have problems, or the next week is hard and I already have it on my mind, I automatically run faster and turn up the music. I can get it out of my system then" (female participant 3).

Isolation by music also allows respondents to disconnect from themselves both physically and mentally, which sometimes shows internal contradictions. Some runners and gym goers pointed out to the need to separate from the sound of their own exertion such as quick and loud breathing as well as the need to turn their attention away from symptoms of weakness described as a "wall":

> "When you have no energy, you can't hear the reaction of your own organism, the deep inhaling and exhaling. That definitely helps overcome weakness" (male participant 4).

While isolating from the signs of tiredness, music reinforces its motivating function, returns or supports the willpower of its users to continue the exercise, and increase endurance levels. At the same time, it isolates on a mental level, facilitating an "escape from reality." The respondents perceived workouts as their time to separate themselves from current life problems, time of solitude, and doing something beneficial for themselves only.

The second essential function of listening to music during a workout stems from its power to model physical activity, which takes place on two levels: directly and indirectly. The direct modeling occurs when listening to music evokes an intense thinking process enabling a workout or making it easier by triggering self-motivation. In that sense, by giving users the "feeling of freedom" and sparking "positive thinking," music increases motivation, puts them in "a better mood in your head," and subsequently makes a workout more pleasant, filling individuals with joy or even happiness:

> "When I hear a song my legs work more energetically. I run with more joy and pleasure" (male participant 1);

> "I can run and run, and I'm happy that I'm running . . ." (female participant 11).

Thus, the power of music to motivate the commencement, continuing, and intensifying physical activity proves its strong indirect modeling power.

Modeling in a direct way derives from music influence on the workout course; on the decisions pertaining to direction and execution. It is closely related to the work of one's own body as the pulse and breathing become synchronized with the rhythm of music:

> "Rhythm synchronizes with the heartbeat, [with] how I breathe. And that becomes compatible with what I'm doing. Music helps me get in tune with myself, with what I'm doing" (male participant 3).

The rhythm and tempo of music are reflected in the rhythm and tempo of movements of a person engaged in physical activity:

"Faster music causes faster movements, faster running" (female participant 4);

"I breathe evenly, my step is even, I have no colic and running is much better" (female participant 10).

Through synchronization with natural body functions and parameters, music becomes its close, natural, adequate, and desirable companion since it models the workout in a manner expected by the listener. It dictates the tempo and synchronizes it with the body:

"It is more a reaction that when I hear it I tune into the rhythm in which everything flows and I feel like synchronizing too" (female participant 11).

Undoubtedly, the deepest modeling sub-process structures a workout or its chosen fragment by music. Examples of that were described by one respondent as "music challenges": workouts where the length of a music piece decides about a certain sequence of movements or a set distance in a particular tempo: "I sprint until the end of this song." That way the music piece or playlist dictates not only the rhythm and tempo of the subsequent movements, but also orders and sequences stages of the entire workout.

Music is expected to enable "putting yourself in the mood for exercise." To achieve that, playlists are often chosen to match a gradual increase in the intensity of a workout. Thus, a mild exercise takes place with songs chosen at random since listening to music seems satisfactory enough and additional mobilization of effort is not necessary. For the purpose of hardest workouts, special "motivating"[19] songs are "reserved," with some respondents categorizing songs praising fight and endurance as "motivating:"

"[When I listen to] epic pieces from battles, when two armies are running one onto another, I can feel the energy buzzing inside me; I could jump, run and do anything (. . .) [it] given me strength" (female participant 11).

The relations between physical activity and listening to music can be described as mutual adjustment. It is evident that strong processual saturation contributes to mediatization seen as the mutual interaction of physical activity and media technologies and processes involved that, inevitably, alter individual training course and regime.

Saturation involving music listening processes trigger three main mechanisms: isolation, modulation, and synchronization. On the one hand, it results in generating pleasure and motivation increase, resulting in turn in a satisfactory completion of a workout, which seems to contribute to the continuity of the taken up exercise. On the other hand, the physical activity leads to selection and evaluation of the chosen playlists, but music does not play an important role in the context of physical activity exclusively; it dictates the rhythm of its user's movement in a broader spectrum. For example, respondents declare that music accompanies them when they "walk around the city" or "are going somewhere," for example:

> "I listen to music almost all the time, when I go from one place to another" (male participant 8).

Music constantly accompanies young users of media technologies and both mobile technology as well as the mediated processes it facilitates become integrated to all users' activities.

Communication

The second mediated process saturating physical activity is based on communication. In the examined case, it takes up three variants: intrapersonal communication, one-to-one, and one-to-many communication. A fourth model can also be distinguished: the lack of any communication during physical activity.

Firstly, it has to be highlighted that in the researched area communication if facilitated by interactive communication[20] mediated by technology. In rare cases, including taking to oneself or conversing with a person accompanying a workout, the intermediary technology is not present.

Intrapersonal Communication

Intrapersonal communication can be defined as communicating with oneself[21] and in physical activity is mediated by verbal and visual messages. It can be illustrated by notes (analog and digital) of which creation and subsequent archiving allow for the analyzing of and a reflection on one's own physical activity: the immediate results, progress made, and future plans. Physical activity becomes a subject of deeply insightful thinking and designing.

The second form of such communication are photos and films created for oneself, e.g., to verify exercise correctness or to observe changes in one's physique. Those materials serve as documentation and are a subject for analysis, but most of all they often become a source of motivation for further activity and its efficient planning.

In rare cases, respondents take photos or videos of the area where they exercise, e.g., beautiful views along the running route. Documenting the surrounding makes the workout more pleasant and allows for the creation of a unique photo or video album to revisit in the future, but it is also a way to converse with oneself during a workout. The place where it takes place is not unimportant as many respondents have their favorite locations, routes, and clubs. Due to the documentation, those locations become even more familiar and they become destinations of not physical workout only, but of a mental process as well.

One-to-one Communication

The rarest, exceptional form of communication during physical activity out of the three aforementioned forms is one-to-one communication. It takes place when a workout is carried out in a company of another person and a conversation occurs. Such situations, however, are not frequent and they are often rated negatively due to their influence on the quality of a workout, with one of the respondents stating that when he runs with another person, he feels like the workout is of a sub-optimal standard.

Such social context forces him to adjust and prevents him from listening to music. Another participant admitted that when she works out in company, she listens to the conversation with one ear while she listens to music with the other and sometimes she gives up music altogether. In her case, conversation served as a substitute for music. Yet another respondent stated that sometimes he calls someone during a run to talk and fill up the time, despite his usual preference for music.

It can be seen, therefore, that a conversation during workout is treated either as a distractor or as a time-filler. Once the workout is completed, asynchronous communication can take place, too. Photos and videos from the workout or taken right after its completion can be sent or posted. Sometimes communication is continued for an extended period of time and is based on exchanging comments on social media about the exercises taken, appearance or exchanging ideas on how to modify the workout in question.

One-to-many Communication

The most diverse form of communication about physical activity is based on the one-to-many model. Two variations can be observed in this case: real-time communication and pre- or post-workout communication. The published content, mainly on social media platforms, is texts, photos, videos of workout routines and surroundings, as well as the achieved results. The dominating aspect observed in that content is the visualization of the respondents' own activity—it seems of paramount importance to show it, not only to describe it.

Therefore, silhouette and weights photos are published as well as videos of gym exercise series. They are most often posted in visual social media such as Instagram and Snapchat, with the latter adding an element of elusiveness to the process of communication since the published photos and videos disappear right after the addressee receives them.[22]

The respondents declare that their preference for Instagram and Snapchat is dictated by a narrow group of recipients, in contrast to much larger potential audience on Facebook. Instagram or Snapchat are therefore seen as communication channels with more selectively chosen public, including mainly closer, more trusted friends and acquaintances who often share interests with the respondents.

Pre- and post-workout communication is done across four social media platforms: Instagram, Snapchat, Facebook, and Tumbler. With the exception of the last one (used by one respondent only), the platforms are used across the sample cohort to a comparable degree and in a similar manner. The users communicate about the achieved results or that the activity has been taken up at all. Some of the respondents favor sharing information about major achievements, beaten records or fair results:

> "Maybe I don't show my workout, but the moment I feel the need, that I did something interesting [sic!]. They are Endomondo results that I put on Facebook" (male participant 1).

Part of the cohort publishes posts illustrating themselves or the context of their workout:

> "It happens that I post something. Everyone wants to show that they're doing something. Everything creates your brand. Once a month I post the distance I achieved, the calories I burnt . . ." (male participant 5).

The importance of self-presentation is underlined by claims that "you should not publish photos that are ugly" or only photos that "look nice and decorate the profile" should be published:

> "[I take the photo] right after the workout. The body is—to use a colloquial term—pumped up the most and looks best" (male participant 4).

Posts are not always limited to a photo or a video only, but sometimes they are accompanied by a description and hashtags, reaching even ten or fifteen in some cases, and this could be dictated by the desire to reach a wider public.

When the context is important to the authors, they record the elements of the environment or their own equipment. It is also an attempt to abstract only the activity, without personalizing it. Such content can include a photo of the time at the run finish line, which eloquently demonstrates the success despite the winner's absence from the image. Similarly, photos of wet shoes and clothing serve as a proof of perseverance, but also an encouragement for others, with the message that "you can run when there's puddles and that it's not an excuse." Motivating others is one of the most often declared reasons for publishing this type of content:

> "It happens to me (that I publish) but not to show off but to motivate myself and others. Often my friends say that they have no energy and that they can't make it. And I ran once, twice and became my lifestyle" (male participant 6).

Some respondents are convinced that sharing such content is highly inspirational:

> "Snapchat is something people receive every moment now. They get info about a photo. They get it every moment and see and think they could try and do something like that too . . ." (male participant 8).

For others, the act of publishing is critically important for the future of their fitness since they perceive it as an expression of commitment:

> "On Instagram, if I say that I'll do something like 1000 push-ups a year and I don't do it, only I will know that. And if I tell others, they will see that. For me that's additional motivation to do what I planned" (male participant 2).

In some cases it actually is a way to inspire external motivation:

> "When someone makes a joke [under the post] that it's "weak," I take it seriously and work out even harder" (male participant 4);

> "Maybe it's like showing off with what I did. So that people would look at me . . ." (male participant 1).

The respondents also indicate other reasons for sharing content, for example, to share the joy of having achieved a target. Many explicitly state that they publish to gain recognition and to draw attention to themselves, to "show themselves," "for fun." Comments and likes are often a source of joy and even deep satisfaction.

Not Publishing—Processual Desaturation

Six out of nineteen respondents do not publish content about their physical activity and are highly critical of such practice. Despite them using media technologies during (and sometimes before and after) training, they neither see the need nor have the desire to share content about themselves, with some participants perceiving that as potentially harmful. In this case, refraining from publishing is an element of the processual desaturation. It pertains to a minority, as the survey results show,[23] but it is a prominent response to widespread media saturation. While for some individuals it is a natural choice, for others it is a direct reaction and response to the surrounding mediatized environment.

A prosaic and rather common argument of those respondents labels sharing as "a waste of time." Communication "gives [them] nothing" and they emphasize that they exercise or run for their own benefit, for health and well-being, and not for others. Therefore, they do not have the need to inform anyone about it.

It seems that respondents have a sense of inadequacy in terms of their content creation skills, stating that others "are better and they have nothing to brag about." Several responses hint at uncertainty or law self-esteem, at times linking sharing with the feeling of shame and embarrassment, unless the achievements comparable to the feat of completing a marathon. A more blatant and recurring stance among those respondents depicts sharing as spamming; in other words, flooding others with meaningless and unsolicited content:

> "I don't want to be a typical teenager; spamming everyone with my workout and annoying everyone" (female participant 11).

Respondents who criticize publishing often point to the need of protecting the "pureness" of physical activity in a somewhat autotelic manner:

> "I don't do fitness because that's a trend. I've been doing it for a long time, before people started going to the gym to take a selfie" (male participant 1);

> "I'm motivated by doing my workout from A to Z and I find taking a photo to show that I'm fit a little off-putting" (female participant 5).

Despite using media technologies that model physical activity, hybridize it, and converge it with other activities; for some respondents nonpublishing serves as a demonstration of resistance to those changes. While monitoring and analyzing data, engaging with media content (mainly music) and the presence of other technologies is acceptable for them, social media sharing evokes opposition and criticism. It is seen as unreasonable, blind trend-following that can be disturbing for their own and others' workouts.

Processual desaturation, in this case labelled as desaturation of publishing processes, is one of the few manifestations of the mediation resistance by individuals who use media technologies. There seems to be a defined boundary between monitoring, data aggregation, analysis, reception of media content, and posting. Those who belong to this group refuse to be prosumers,[24] co-authors of media content about their own activity, and are staunch critics of social media sharing.

Self-tracking and Other Mediated Processes

It is evident that real-time analysis of exercise parameters directly determines the course of a workout. In this context, technological saturation is characterized by close integration of human physical activity and monitoring as well as analytical activity of a sport tracker or other controlling device. Prior to digital technology expansion, it could be observed at gyms among people using exercise machines (treadmills, stationary training bikes, etc.) equipped with basic measuring tools. Currently, technological saturation is possible regardless of training location or stationary equipment accessibility and its range has significantly widened.

More importantly, data archiving allows, in the words of one participant, to "gather history." The next stage is data manipulation based on statistical studies within individual and collective dimension. This enhances the importance of monitoring and justifies it to a certain extent, provided that it is accompanied by analysis in a numerical, descriptive, or visual form.

Some commonly archived and analyzed elements are routes that runners are eager to revisit. The data visualization on maps, for examples, allows participants to trace a route, return to it, and analyze its geographical features, such as its incline, altitude changes, etc. An application enables users to visualize not only the route, but, in a sense, the workout, too. The physical experience during the activity is depicted and recorded, and it has gained the qualities of evidence, or a keepsake, and often advice for the future.

Endomondo, most commonly used, provides advanced numerical analyses used for the needs of future workouts. The respondents seem mostly interested in the training evolution over time in relation to recorded parameters. Some claim it equips them with knowledge about a training element they need to improve. Saturation with analytical processes bears, therefore, long-term importance. It affects not only the present workout, but it models its future shape, with subsequent training sessions determined by the received data sets and recommendations. This arises both out of the hard data that the users take into account, and also from its purely motivational function, as respondents unanimously strive for their consecutive results to be better than the last and for meeting their individual targets.

Endomondo also serves a source of social evidence for the completed activity and the achieved results. Through integration with social media, it enables real-time and post-factum sharing of, for example, formatted posts with results "endorsed" by Endomondo. Quite unsurprisingly, the respondents favor sharing their personal records and other special achievements with the automatic post generated by Endomondo via, i.e., Facebook serving as a validation of their achievements. Thus, posting becomes a source of additional satisfaction and motivation, with trackers playing an important role in that process, however, they are not the only means facilitating that.

An example within the context of motivational function, but also providing diversification, is the Pokemon Go mobile app. To one user, a gamified run proved to be a source of enhanced satisfaction, providing symbolic rewards for the effort she made. The game tokens stimulated her motivation for achievement and made her feel elated upon obtaining them.

While it did not exclude potential disappointment with the run or the results of the game, the continuation of the physical activity (in this case the run) offered the possibility of reliving the elation, enhanced in conjunction with the satisfaction of the distance traveled:

"I can grow an egg during a run for 2, 5 or 10 kilometers. It's simple, you get information, wow, you ran 5 km and it's great, but here when you run 5 km you have another wow—a Pokemon that hatched from the egg. It's a reward for your running (. . .). It was great when Pikachu popped out. I was happy because I didn't have it. It's worse when I already have the thing that pops out. I'm not so happy then. But what can you do, I drop another egg into the incubator and run on" (female participant 11).

The physical activity in this case has taken a particularly hybrid character. It both demands physical effort and offers a game-play, strongly saturated with mediated processes, including content creation as the respondent generated images deriving from her multidimensional activity. Since she used media technology for a variety of purposes, her workouts became more attractive and unique in that respect.

PHYSICAL ACTIVITY AND
MEDIA TECHNOLOGY PREFERENCES

Factors

To further examine mediated processes, the study investigated specifics of the processual saturation of physical activity, including decisive factors for the preference of particular sport and their correlation with the chosen media technologies.

To address this point, respondents' statements defining their key reasons and factors influencing physical activity choice were subjected to detailed analysis and categorization. This led to identification of co-deciding factors that can be broadly divided into the following categories:

• body-oriented and mind-oriented,
• self-oriented and others-oriented.

The division is rather typical, and while indirect categories can also be distinguished, the main orientation of the described activity (body/mind, self/others) captures its hybrid, convergent nature, which acquires new features due to media saturation.

Body-oriented factors refer to the needs and reasons behind the choice of an activity aimed at achieving particular effects within or outside the body. These factors are described as "strengthening the whole body," "taking care of the body," working on "body aesthetics," doing "something for the body," "learning your organism," "growing muscle," express the need to "manage your body," and "maintaining weight."

Some of them address the physiological or wider biological processes that the human body undergoes. Those include: "getting enough oxygen," improving appearance and silhouette, increasing fitness, endurance, stamina, recovering from an injury, obtaining or even getting rid of energy excess, acquiring competence for self-defense, improving sleep quality, health, enhancing diet effects, getting rid of physical pain, or even achieving post-workout fatigue.

Predictably, mind-oriented factors refer to psyche and intellect, including mood, emotions, affectation, and cognitive aspects. The desire to feel better, to pursue passion, to do something beneficial for oneself, and to achieve a sense of pride and fulfillment have been commonly listed by the participants. At the same time, they also expressed a sense of duty, particularly toward themselves. This is captured by statements referring to "doing something for yourself," "doing something useful," "working on yourself," "doing your best," with the emphasis on perseverance, permanence, being systematic, and even "working on your own character." For some participants, a completed workout guarantees inner peace for the entire day, and hence they prefer to pursue their training regime in the morning. Often the reasons behind engaging in physical activity stem from the pursuit of change and challenge: "defeating oneself/your own weaknesses," "being a better copy of oneself," "liking yourself."

Some factors are of a social nature and thus they are oriented toward others. They serve a social function (the opportunity to meet or just be among other people), facilitate self-presentation ("show others that I can do something"), demonstrate a sense of fashion (surrender to being "fit"), or a response to social pressure ("I did it only because everyone else did it"). Other-oriented seem much less prevalent, which suggests that physical activity primarily stems from the respondents' own needs (and not the needs of others), and that those needs are mostly fulfilled in solitude.[25]

Among the mind-oriented factors, the dominating tendency is to "escape from reality," "to break away from daily life/daily duties," the pursuit of "thinking only about running—nothing else." In that context, physical activity facilitates the opportunity to "work it off," "chill out," "calm down," compose oneself, find the "time to think," "time only for yourself," being "alone with one's thoughts," and finally, to gain a sense of freedom:

> "[What is it that running gives you the most?]
> That I can compose myself. I am alone with my own thoughts. Nobody tells me where to run. And it gives me that freedom" (male participant 6).

Almost half of the interviewees refer to the need for isolation in a straightforward manner while the statements of several others are indirectly linked to the stress-relieving and therapeutic aspects of physical activity.

From the perspective of the studied discourse, including both statements content and the manner of their expression, the mind-oriented factors strongly dominate over the body-oriented determinants. The former appears in statements more often[26] and are of a more elaborate and personalized nature.

Patterns

Escape

The mind-oriented factors, which are mainly self-oriented (especially illustrated by the common tendency to isolate oneself), correspond strongly with the processes of listening to music, which also serves as an isolator. In the examined group of runners and gym goers, it is the most important process modeling physical activity, even when it is simultaneously accompanied by tracking with, e.g., Endomondo, or by interpersonal communication. Physical activity, therefore, appears to be facilitating solitude, and developing a mental enclave, generally inaccessible to others.

This can occur through strong technological saturation, facilitated by the permanent use of earphones intersected with processual saturation seen as the saturation of physical activity with listening to music. Through its modeling, synchronizing, and above all, isolating, impact, the physical activity is transformed into a separating activity. This is supported by the respondents, perceiving physical activity as the time of separation, both in material, physical, and visibility sense as well as in its nonmaterial and purely mental aspect.

Therefore, the purpose of physical activity accompanied by music is, to an extent, the attainment of a particular state of mind rather than the specific state of the body. Understandably, long-term effects do affect the biological and mental sphere, but technological and processual saturation play such an important role mainly due to their immediacy. As such, it is revealing that none of the interviewees linked listening to music to achieving certain biological effects, although music indirectly plays an important role in that context.

The above pattern of physical activity with the use of media technology (in this case an audio technology) can be defined as an escape or separation pattern. Hybrid activity, combining motion and media, is aimed at isolation, a separation in the material and nonmaterial dimension.

Effects

Another pattern emerging from the respondents' statements is the focus on the effects. This pattern is strongly correlated with body-oriented goals, which, as indicated earlier, are prevalent among the minority but of chief importance in this context. The focus on the effects leads to strict data monitoring and analysis to ensure maximum efficiency in terms of distance, time, weight, number of repetitions, etc. Without digital media technology (and in rare cases analog technology), achieving the desired effects can be more challenging and lack of direct application-based data can deem validating a particular goal impossible in some cases. In other circumstances, accepting certain assumptions is a key determinant for the course and success of training. In many cases, however, the absence of technology undermines these assumptions and thus assessing whether set targets have been met is impossible. Sometimes, accepting certain assumptions, completely determines the course and the end of training. In many cases, without the use of media technologies, confirmation that the target has been achieved is impossible.

> "I try to demand a 100 percent from myself. I do not finish a cardio workout if I don't burn 300 calories" (male participant 2).

The focus on maximizing the effects corresponds with the long-term impact of physical activity, aided by the use of media technologies. As demonstrated earlier, media technologies have the potential to model it for the purposes of efficiency, which in turn contributes to maintaining continuity:

> "The more you exercise, the more effects you see. And that drives you to work out even harder" (male participant 3).

In the long run, the effects are monitored by tracking various parameters, such as progress, distribution of effects over time, body weight, and other measurements. Users also monitor their own appearance and changes in silhouette, for example, by taking pictures. For some interviewees, satisfaction and well-being are determined by good results across those parameters and physical activity effectiveness evidenced by technology (mostly from mobile applications, but also photos and videos) reinforces their sense of satisfaction.

Within the context of focusing on the effects, the importance of media saturation is not as much related to the present moment as to the long-term impact of many factors, including media saturation on physical activity of individuals.

Pleasure

The most rarely occurring pattern refers to running and working out for pleasure. Some respondents state that without feeling pleasure, physical activity makes no sense and can quickly lead to its termination:

> "Sport is healthy, you meet new friends, but it needs to give you pleasure. Otherwise, it's just a one or two months adventure . . ." (male participant 2).

This pleasure may be different in its character. It can involve the biologically sensed change in the body (secretion of endorphins) as well as the previously described sense of satisfaction deriving from performing a useful activity or leading to a sense of fulfillment. Some respondents directly indicate that physical activity and music combined give them the greatest pleasure in life. That integration influences the human body and the psyche to a great extent and the impact of media technologies can be observed.

The three patterns described above are ideal types and in practice they intertwine. The escape pattern, however, predominates and is accompanied by the mindset focused on efficiency or pleasure, or both simultaneously.

Contradictions

Based on the research, the emerging image of runners and gym goers who listen to music and use other media technologies is homogeneous and devoid of contradictions. That pertains to both physical activity and the importance of media technology involved. During the interviews, less than one-third of the interviewees contradicted themselves, which may indicate that they were not entirely sincere. This may have been caused by the reluctance to disclose all details of their thoughts, problems they are often unaware of, or insecurity and timidity.

It may also have resulted from the lack of complete awareness of the processes that the respondents were implementing and that they were subjected to.[27] In some cases, the contradictions indicate that young, physically active people are subjected to multidimensional pressures, both internally and externally. It would not be folly to conclude, therefore, that they try to meet particular social pressures through media saturation, and subsequent individualization and modeling of physical activity, while remaining as free as possible.

The main contradiction observed refers to the described escape mechanism. Runners and gym goers want to separate themselves in different dimensions and via varied means. They strive to break away from the reality not related to their workout, yet, they spend their training time pondering over issues that are not relevant to their workout. They claim that this is a relaxation time, yet they focus on their problems. They analyze, plan, meditate—not necessarily about pleasant matters:

"It's definitely time to think over everyday issues, to plan the next day. It's a form of relaxation and staying in shape" (male participant 5);

"I can be with my workout, with my problems. I think about them during my workout" (female participant 4).

In that process, music plays a variety of functions: it is supposed to calm one down, but can also act as a driver; in other words, it can be used to compose oneself or evoke emotions, add energy, and relieve of energy. While in some cases it is supposed to help break away from one's thoughts, in others the aim is to aid the thinking process. Regardless of the end goal, it can be concluded that the time spent working out with music acts as catharsis—it purifies one from current issues, both intellectually and emotionally.

However, one can get the impression that, despite the fact that young people strive to achieve general stability in life through training, they do not use all available technological and exercise resources for that purpose. Their reflections on the desire to enjoy physical activity are followed by those stressing the need to find a way for completing their activities in shorter time frames. At times, they experience inner emptiness while exercising and they try to fill it in with music and other audio content: radio programs, audiobooks, or television, or just "some sounds."

Physical activity, despite some respondents' declarations, is not a pleasure in itself, and music facilitates another sort of an escape: from the overwhelming aspects of training. Music as a source of pleasure and training modulator becomes a "jammer" of one's own body; a tool for self-deception. Fitness enthusiasts embark on an activity targeting their own body, but at the same time they isolate themselves from it. Hearing the sounds of their within, their own bodies or their breath is not desirable, and music can shield from that. A similar function is played by interpersonal communication. The same individuals who declare they do not talk to anyone to focus on training at other times admit that they deliberately make phone calls while running to make their activity pleasant (which is otherwise experienced as sub-standard or hard).

Contradictions also relate to the desire to improve one's well-being. It is one of the chief reasons for engaging in physical activity, but it is accompanied by intrinsic pressure of both an internal and external nature, undertake that activity, and to achieve particular results. In the absence of progress or the presumed pleasure from the workout, a sense of guilt appears. A workout becomes a morning chore undertaken "to have it over with." Not surprisingly, therefore, anticipating a workout is sometimes seen as tiring and a burden:

"If I don't run I feel like I haven't done anything for myself, for my own pleasure . . ." (male participant 5).

One of the most frequently encountered contradictions lies in the attitude toward numerical results and posting about physical activity. In the former case, results are often trivialized and described as meaningless. In the course of a conversation, however, it turns out that respondents use a sport tracker application and are fully aware of the data collected and their own results, providing the total number of kilometers run, the average monthly distance, etc. This clearly indicates the importance of the achieved results, only seemingly disregarded by the respondents.

Similarly, the criticism of posting activities is often accompanied by admitting such conduct. Even when content of this kind is judged as tiresome (for others and the respondents themselves), it eventually transpires that the desire to present their activity is stronger than the possibility of a negative judgment by their peers. However, it is important to emphasize that both internal and external pressure to be present on social media does not affect all of the respondents.

Excluding the impact of possible embarrassment (deriving from being self-conscious about bragging on the Internet) on the respondents' honesty, it is evident that not all participants are fully aware of what aids or hinders their physical activity. Above all, they do not seem to be conscious of the role media technologies can play in that process. Some respondents even try to devaluate media technologies, which is not reflected in their practice. It is best illustrated by a male interviewee categorically stating that "no technology can help. What counts is the effort and that's it," followed by his admission that he scrupulously records all the results of his training sessions, watches

instructional videos, listens to music while exercising, and uses various measuring devices at the gym to verify "if his workout makes sense at all."

Through intensive structural and processual saturation, media technologies
become not only transparent and natural, so that their presence and usage are
unnoticeable, but their direct impact on individuals became inconspicuous.
This is one of the main implications of media saturation, which arises from
the high degree of saturation, both in the individual and social dimension.
Media technologies are ubiquitous in peoples' lives and their environment
and they no longer evoke much interest or fear, resulting from the effects of
their presence and usage. In addition, using technology is a highly hybrid activity, requiring to enter into deep relationships with numerous processes and
mechanisms, both on a social and psychological level, through which they
co-model their users' lives. They become supportive, needed, and at times,
absolutely indispensable.

Mediatization of Dominating Forms of Physical Activity

In the context of the analyzed data focusing on the audio and self-tracking
technologies, it should be emphasized that the results both confirm several
general conclusions as well as supplement or revise the meaning of particular
phenomena or processes.

Listening to Music

Listening to music appeared to be the most important mediated process that
saturates physical activity in the investigated cohort and it is a subject of
research of physical activity scientists and psychologists too. The hitherto
conducted research mainly pertains to the psychological effects of mediated
processes in terms of mood, emotions, affection (feeling pleasure), cognition,
and behavior. The analysis of psycho-physical effects (specified sometimes
as psycho-physiological) refers to physiological changes that result from
listening to music during a workout, including blood pressure increase, the
pulse change, etc. In addition, the ergogenic effects pertain to increased endurance, including stamina, strength, productivity, etc.

While the research results inscribe into the statements made in previous
sections, particularly in terms of psychological and ergogenic effects, they
also bring in new elements of high importance.

From the perspective of the conceptual model by Costas I. Karageorghis
and Peter C. Terry, the meaning of initial factors was confirmed in the case
of amateurs: both in their personal (like mood) and circumstantial (like other
people being present during the workout, etc.) dimensions. The meaning of

rhythm,[28] musicality,[29] and cultural meaning[30] of music listened to during a workout was examined and categorized against the model. The analysis showed a similar set of benefits that users gain from listening to music during physical activity, including improved mood, controlled stimulation, and higher efficiency.[31]

The synchronous, asynchronous, and *pre-task* use of music singled out by P. C. Terry and I. Karageorghis is also reflected in the presented results. The mechanism of structurization is present, but not limited to synchronizing function of music; the pleasing functions refer to asynchronizing and pre-task motivational action.

The analysis of media saturation addresses a gap in research on the meaning of processes and benefits deriving from the use of media technologies, in both material and processual dimension. The importance of physical presence of media technologies e.g., in or on the body of an exercising individual or in their immediate and distant surrounding appeared. Also, the significance of the listening technology (e.g., in helping sportspeople "to cocoon themselves in their own audio world,"[32]) was confirmed in the studied cohort of amateurs and the meaning of personalized music playlists was also examined. [33]

The research that was undertaken significantly supplements the hitherto published studies on the importance of audio technologies. Such research, is often positioned at the intersection of urban studies, cultural studies, and sociology, which are dominated by the analysis of the usage of audio technologies in city space and, according to Michael Bull, focus on "visual epistemology of experience rather than an auditory one" with more "externalist" than "internalist" approach.[34] The three dimensions, categorized by M. Bull as "relational experience" divided between cognitive, aesthetic, and moral dimensions,[35] explicitly require to be supplemented by yet another element: the bodily one, pertaining to movement and physical activity. The users not only "transform or control their mood, thoughts and forms of interaction with others and their environment," but also alter the course of their physical activity. M. Bull considers this strategy to play an energizing function, resulting in "body work[ing] in rhythm to the music."[36] As the results of the media saturation analysis indicate, modification is a highly complex process. For example, in the context of movement, one does not gain control from listening to music, but renounces it, allowing for the music to modulate the activity. Similarly, acoustic separation serves users not only to isolate from other people or surrounding sounds, but to cut off from themselves (e.g., their loud breathing, etc.).

The modification described by M. Bull of, for example, the work that one does in the context of physical activity occurs on a different level: a physical level with emotions and socio-cultural experiences both internal and external modulated. The mediatized physical activity is characterized by other processes across various dimensions taking place concurrently. Subordinating thoughts and emotions, in other words, "sorting yourself and the entire world," can occur on dual level: during physical exercise and sometimes through them. There are, however, many similarities between using audio technologies in the city space, as indicated by M. Bull, and during physical activity. These include, but are not limited to the importance of a playlist, personalization of music and the importance of sourcing new tunes, limiting the feeling of wasting one's time, facilitating better focus, and creating "music challenges" for oneself.

Sport Self-tracking

Due to a relative novelty of self-tracking technologies and services (compared with, e.g., portable music players), studies on those devices are a rather new area. The hitherto published research, therefore, located within the strand categorized as life-logging, personal analytics, quantified self, mainly pertains to monitoring and analyzing health condition,[37] with sport self-trackers remaining a much less investigated area. However, there are some similarities in research results obtained to date. For example, Stine Lombork and Kirsten Frandsen indicate that using sport trackers integrates the individual and social dimension (meaning "performing oneself, and upholding a set of social relations"[38]) and, to a large extent, it is conditioned by affordances of the used technologies, which is analyzed in depth by the saturation studies presented in this volume. The media saturation studies explain further the importance of pleasure and effectiveness in physical activity, which are also mentioned by S. Lomborg and K. Frandsen. In addition, they indicate the change mechanisms "from a bodily experience into a psychological experience,"[39] with the emphasis on the patterns of physical activity and the resulting contradictions, rather than merely on the fusion of contemplativeness and flexible routines.[40] Lastly, studies carried out by both authors demonstrate similar motivating functions (self-motivation and external motivation). It is contradictory to the conclusions of John Rooksby et.all,[41] stating that tracking is a social rather than an individual phenomenon. The results obtained refute those conclusions while they confirm the importance of technologies in creating documentation and specifying short-term and long-term goals.[42] Similarly, on the structural level, they accentuate the difficulties arising from the devices being unhandy, the risk of losing them, or the necessity to remember to carry the device, turning it on or having to enter data manually,[43] which further confirms that devices remain nonperfect in terms of their design and functionality.

MEDIA SATURATION INVESTIGATION

The results of the research of the sport-media worlds of runners and gym goers affected by the use of music players and other media technologies demonstrate that the quality of the technological saturation and processual saturation is very complex and multidimensional. Within the research context, the specifics of technological saturation are the result of the construction, the design, and affordances particular to smartphones and, to a lesser extent, to other technologies. The distinctive nature of the processual saturation is based mainly on receiving, tracking, and diversifying processes.

Due to the combination of both dimensions of saturation, the basic mechanisms of mediatization were revealed. They emerged from the analysis of relations between quantitative and qualitative properties of the devices and their operation in activity. The main mechanisms observed in the researched group were of an individual or social nature.

The analysis confirmed and underlined the necessity to adapt a nonmedia-centric perspective. The diversity of processes into which media technologies are incorporated is too wide and complex to perceive technologies as the main drivers of change. The psychological and physiological needs of individuals, social trends and fashion, as well as economic and logistic accessibility of both technology and sports, play an important role.

Integrating the material and symbolic perspectives in the analysis of the media technologies role in physical activity revealed the dual nature of mediatization. Mediatization does not occur exclusively as a result of social communication on and within a given area, but above all, as a result of technology-mediated processes based on communicating with the devices. To a great extent, mediatization processes occur due to the material properties of media technology that remain independent of their content. Whether their content comprises of a telephone conversation, a radio program, an audiobook or music, the unchanging element lies in the importance of using earphones and opening adequate applications that presence explicitly conditions physical activity commencement. Undoubtedly, the conjured picture is not devoid of flaws, dissonances, or contradictions. However, the quantitative measurement of the degree and spectrum of saturation combined with the qualitative analysis of the mechanisms' density, allows to distinguish original patterns of media saturation, and ipso facto the mechanisms of mediatization.

NOTES

1. The research was conducted between September and November 2016.
2. Wrocław agglomeration was selected again.
3. The number of interviews is similar to qualitative research in that area, e.g., Lomborg and Frandsen (twelve people), Rooksby et.al (twenty-two people). Stine

Lomborg and Kirsten Frandsen, "Self-tracking as Communication," *Information, Communication & Society* 19.7 (2016); John Rooksby et al., "Personal Tracking as Lived Informatics," *Proceedings of the 32nd Annual ACM Conference on Human Factors in Computing Systems* (ACM, 2014).

4. More in chapter 1.

5. Only one respondent delivered a photo with headphones visible.

6. The details pertaining to isolation from the surroundings are described further in the chapter.

7. The meaning of music in a workout is described in detail further in the chapter.

8. More details in the section devoted to processual saturation.

9. Desaturation of physical activity is described in chapter 5.

10. More on contradictions can be found further in the volume.

11. This technology group is complemented by internet services, i.e., focused on diets (such as calorie calculators). While they are not directly dedicated to physical activity, they are an additional element and supplement the technologies by aspects that are important for the respondents in their physical activity.

12. The analog pedometer mentioned before.

13. Details can be found further in the volume.

14. For example, one respondent stated that when she plans a run under 5 km, she does not listen to music: "by the time I hook up the equipment I can run that distance."

15. One respondent stated that knowing that he will exercise at the gym in a company, he does not even bring his music player with him.

16. In this case it is most often a result of forgetting to bring the equipment or depleted battery.

17. The respondents listed: hip hop, heavy metal, jazz, dub step, rap, film soundtracks, rock, pop, relaxation music, reggae, dance music, techno, classical music, and other kinds.

18. Mainly disco-polo (simple, popular music in Poland).

19. According to one of the interviewers, a good example of such music is Eminem's song "Lose Yourself" from the movie *Eight Mile*.

20. Friedrich Krotz, "Media as a Societal Structure and a Situational Frame for Communicative Action: A Definition of Concepts," in *Critical Perspectives on the European Mediasphere*, eds. Ilija Tomanić Trivundža, Nico Carpentier, Hannu Nieminen, Pille Pruulmann-Venerfeldt, Richard Kilborn, Ebba Sundin and Tobias Olsson (Lubljana: Faculty of Social Sciences: Založba FDV, 2011): 36.

21. "Intrapersonal communication refers to the creating, functioning, and evaluating of symbolic processes which operate primarily within oneself. Levels of intrapersonal communication range along a continuum according to the extent messages are stored in the environment around the self-communicating system. Such activities as "thinking," "mediating," and "reflecting," which may require no environmental storage outside the life space of the communicator, are on one end of this continuum and activities such as "talking aloud to oneself" and "writing oneself a note," which require considerably more environmental storage, are on the other end of this continuum," Larry L. Barker, and Gordon Wiseman, "A Model of Intrapersonal Communication," *Journal of Communication* 16.3 (1966): 173.

22. There is a possibility to play the message within twenty-four hours of receiving it, but then it permanently disappears.

23. See chapter 2.

24. Alvin Toffler, *The Third Wave* (New York: Bantam Books, 1980).

25. Clearly, a category of intermediate factors could be distinguished and those are located between self-orientation and orientation toward others, but they are included in the body-oriented category.

26. Only one respondent showed stronger orientation toward the body, which might have come from an external, utilitarian motivation as she was training to be accepted in the military services. Two other participants demonstrated a balanced orientation toward body and mind as their statements comprised of an even number of factors of both types.

27. This may be related to the relatively young age of the respondents.

28. Rhythm response: mainly reaction to tempo (the speed of music counted in bits per minute); Costas I. Karageorghis and Peter C. Terry, "Psychophysical Effects of Music in Sport and Exercise: An Update on Theory, Research and Application," in *Proceedings of the 2006 Joint Conference of the Australian Psychological Society and New Zealand Psychological Society* (Auckland: Australian Psychological Society, 2006): 415.

29. Mainly elements such as harmony, melody. Ibid., 415.

30. Cultural impact: references to social and cultural sphere. Ibid.

31. Ibid., 416.

32. Costas I. Karageorghis and Peter C. Terry, "The Psychological, Psychophysical, and Ergogenic Effects of Music in Sport: A Review and Synthesis," in *Sporting Sounds: Relationships Between Sport and Music*, eds. Anthony Bateman and John Bale (London: Routledge, 2009), 13.

33. Like in previous research e.g.: "(. . .) interventions including self-selected music and imagery could enhance athletic performance by triggering emotions and cognitions associated with flow. (. . .) self-selected music enhanced perceptions of state self-confidence." Costas and Terry, *Psychophysical Effects* . . ., 418. The role of media technologies that enable pre-task selection and real-time selection of playlists requires deeper analysis. Also, the meaning of other functionalities and affordances require additional specification and the relationships between audio technologies used and the remaining media—sometimes integrated—technologies necessitate particular attention.

34. Michael Bull, "Investigating the Culture of Mobile Listening: From Walkman do iPod," in *Consuming Music Together: Social Collaborative Aspects of Music Consumption Technologies*, eds. Kenton O'Hara and Barry Brown (Heidelberg: Springer 2006), 134.

35. Ibid., 133.

36. Ibid., 135.

37. Lomborg and Frandsen, ibid. 1015–1027.

38. Ibid., 10.

39. Ibid., 1022.

40. Ibid., 1019.

41. Rooksby et.al., ibid.,1163

42. Ibid.

43. Ibid.,1167.

Chapter Four

Qualitative Measurement of Media Saturation of Physical Activity

Niche Forms of Physical Activity and Niche Technologies

Aimed at grasping the mechanisms of physical activity mediatization, the qualitative study of media saturation does not only require the examination of dominating technologies and forms of physical activity (and the relationships between them), but also a deeper insight into the properties of their relatively niche alternatives. It is dictated by the need to assess whether physical activity mediatization mechanisms occur in a similar manner in both cases and draw comparatives between saturation with universal and popular technologies as opposed to specialist and niche technologies. Similarly, it serves as a test for the hypothesis that popular forms of physical activity (like running and gym workouts) show different qualitative features of saturation to sports activities favored by only a small number of individuals. It is also essential to examine the relationship between niche sports and widely-used media technology forms.

The survey carried out for the purpose of this study revealed that personal video cameras (built-in smartphone cameras[1] and independent, GoPro[2]-type cameras) were relatively seldom used in niche sports disciplines. It showed that only a small percentage of individuals, who mainly engage in most popular forms of physical activity (e.g., running and gym workout), use personal video cameras[3] and these technologies more often find use in less popular and niche activities.

The rationale behind research on the processes related to filming one's own physical activity is based on several observations.

Following devices and applications used for listening to music, radio, watching TV or films, or self-tracking, video camera is the most common technology listed by the respondents. Researching it, therefore, enables to grasp the mechanisms typical for mediated processes than facilitate communication (such as listening, and mainly publishing processes depicted so far) and monitoring as well as data analyzing.

In addition, video-taping is the second most often selected form of individual, non-automatic and audio-visual recording of one's own physical activity (after photo-taking). Also, video cameras are used by individuals engaging in a variety of sport disciplines, including outdoor and indoor activities, which leads to usage diversification. Moreover, it faces less limitations compared to niche technologies, such as augmented reality or Kinect-type games.

Based on the survey, the aims of using video cameras in physical activity vary. They include satisfaction goals such as:

- effectiveness (getting better sport results),
- multitasking (e.g., the ability to perform a few activities simultaneously),
- tracking (monitoring, analysis, and archiving data of physical activity) to modify activity during its course and reinforcing its effects (aimed at health improvement and appearance enhancements),
- socio-cultural activities (e.g., sharing of the results with others).

It can be seen, therefore, that video recording affects many areas of everyday life and the following sections offer an in-depth examination of its governing processes in the context of visual communication and the growing popularity of audio-visual content on social media platforms.

The analysis of the collected data pertaining to the forms of activity[4] allowed for a selection of those considered niche due to the following (yet not necessarily concurrent) reasons:

- They are poorly known activities; emerging and/or not widely propagated,
- They require a rare set of skills and characteristics combined, e.g., courage, extreme stamina and condition, patience and consistency, etc.
- They are disciplines, sub-disciplines, or variants of activities carried out only in specific, uncommon conditions (e.g., terrain or weather conditions), that condition their uniqueness,
- They require substantial financial resources than most common disciplines.

Fourteen forms of physical activity were chosen, including cross-fit, calisthenics, fitness body building, paragliding, skiing, rowing, classic horse riding, western style horse riding, pole dance, MMA, figure rollerblading, ballroom dancing, parkour, and mountain biking.

They were selected based on their contrasting characteristics that allowed for a proportionate comparison to be made (with the general assumptions when defining them):[5]

- outdoor (eight) and indoor (six) activities,
- seasonal (seven) and all-year-round (seven) activities,[6]
- emerging (eight) and well-established (six) activities,
- relatively low-cost activities that do not require specialist equipment and conditions (seven) and high-cost disciplines requiring specialist equipment and conditions (seven).

Based on the above selection criteria, a cross-section of diverse forms of physical activities was distinguished, which enabled for a wider and a more in-depth examination of the specifics of niche sports media saturation.

The sample included seven women and seven men aged between 21 and 34 years, with the average age of 29. The omission of the youngest group (15–20 years old) and the inclusion of the remaining number of older individuals from the preceding survey was dictated by the following factors:

- the survey results showed that more individuals aged 19–24 (than those between 15–18) declared the use of a GoPro camera and smartphone cameras to communication purposes (e.g., creating media content later posted on social media) during physical activity,
- individuals aged between 21 and 34 have a potentially larger budget, allowing for the investment in less common, though more costly forms of physical activity,
- compared to 15–18-year-olds, those aged between 21 and 34 are more likely to engage in physical activity to a greater extent, potentially leading to higher levels of advancement in their sport discipline, which may translate into a more significant investment of time and resources, including media technologies,
- older individuals are more likely to professionalize their physical activity resulting from the opportunity to pursuit profiting from that, which in turn may trigger a tendency to use media technologies supporting professionalization.

Based on the above discussion on sample characteristics, there were seven individuals practicing entirely amateur physical activities (including paragliding, MMA, skiing, figure skating, parkour, rowing, and western horse riding), six who treated sport as a source of income (cross-fit, calisthenics, body building, mountain biking, pole dance, and ballroom dancing), and one participant in the process of their physical activity commercialization (classic horse riding).

It is important to note that the participants cannot be classified as professionals since they do not gain substantial profits from participating in competitions, but generate incentives from, for example, the coaching or advisory services they render. Thus, their own physical activity strengthens their value as professionals in the broadly defined sports industry. Sport, therefore, serves as their additional income source, not limited to its practice and taking part in subsequent competitions. Training and competitions serve only a base, a starting point for earning money within sport services (as a trainer, instructor, consultant, etc.) or through endorsement activities such as advertising of sports products. It is also worth noting that the researched non-amateurs, who can be described as paraprofessionals,[7] represent different sport disciplines in terms of their status.[8] For example, cross-fit, parkour, and figure rollerblading are not perceived as qualified disciplines, i.e., those where formal competitions take place under a supervision of an association created for the needs of a given sport.[9] However, fitness bodybuilding, a variation of traditional bodybuilding, is seen as a fully qualified sport, since relevant sports associations supervise organizational issues related to practicing that discipline. Similarly, mountain biking and classic horse riding are qualified sports, with the western-style horse riding in the process of becoming one. Quite on a different end of the spectrum is ballroom dancing: it is recognized as a nonsport and considered to be a form of recreation.

Sample participants were selected based on the following criteria:

- practicing sport regularly (at least once a week and for a minimum of sixty minutes a week),
- using personal cameras (built into a smartphone or independent, GoPro-type) during physical activity, alone or in a company.

Since all respondents declared engagement in more than one form of physical activity, the cohort was diversified in many aspects. In terms of the specificity of a given form of activity as well as the conditions required to practice it, the sample represented a wide array of goals underlining physical activity (commercial or noncommercial character). Also, it included older individuals, who have not been present in the hitherto examined samples.

In order to determine the specifics of media saturation in niche forms of physical activity, integrated research methods of fourteen cases were used:[10]

- individual, in-depth, semi-structured interview,
- survey questionnaire,
- observation (including analysis of video recordings and photos taken during the observations), and/or analysis of visual materials and other data provided by the respondents (photos, videos, statistics from mobile application reports).[11]

TECHNOLOGICAL SATURATION

Smartphonization Through Video Recording

In the investigated cohort, the vast majority of respondents (thirteen out of fourteen individuals)[12] use cameras built into their smartphones for the process of video recording their physical activity. In addition, five individuals alternate between or simultaneously use other cameras (GoPro and other digital cameras), while ten out of fourteen respondents make recordings individually. While recording, only a minority keeps the smartphone in hand or mounted on oneself, either attached to clothing, to accessories (e.g., on a helmet), or accompanying equipment (e.g., harness of a paraglider). However, the majority of individuals position the smartphone at a distance from themselves to achieve a certain perspective. One third of the respondents get recorded by a third party, which results from the specificity of their discipline. This applies to western-style horse riding, MMA, and rowing. Those activities require frequent position changes combined with movement and this significantly increases the risk of causing damage to the devices. Therefore, presence and participation of a filming person is necessary (e.g., a trainer or a helmsman). Occasionally, some respondents use the help of others, including training partners, purely to be able to view their own performance from a different point of view (mountain biking, figure rollerblading, fitness body building).

Constellation of Media Technologies

Smartphone is positioned at the core of media technologies constellation of the researched sports enthusiasts. However, apart from a built-in camera enabling high-quality photos and videos, this device is expected to be compatible with other devices, including speakers (portable and stationary, available, e.g., at a gym) and applications (mainly social media apps) were photo and video materials that aid their close integration with the course of the exercise (including preparation and post-recovery). Such constellations include software technologies (applications) and devices (stationary and mobile). The average number of technologies used in physical activity by the respondents was five, with the maximum reaching eight.

Unsurprisingly, recording with a built-in camera built entails the use of other technologies, i.e., video editing applications, social websites where the videos are published, and often loudspeakers playing music, which simultaneously serves as a soundtrack to the created video. At the same time, other technologies integrated with the smartphone are launched (sport trackers, maps, messengers) during the course of the said exercise.

Clearly, independent technologies are located outside of the network of technologies converging with smartphones. Often, they are not integrated with smartphones (i.e., standalone music players, navigation devices, on-board computers, heart-rate monitors), and some operate in an entirely independent manner (wall timers, watches, stopwatches, trainers built into training devices, TV sets, independent cameras, and video cameras).

Individuals engaging in niche sports use specialized media technologies dedicated to their chosen disciplines, but those technologies constitute a minority (applications for cyclists, paragliders, skiers; on-board computers, navigation devices). Universal devices (social media apps, music players) and technologies (sport trackers, heart rate monitors, electronic trainers) are still most widely used.

The technology constellations arranged by the individuals engaging in sports are very diverse. Each discipline shows its specificity where those are further modified by their users' preferences. However, the common use of two technologies—smartphones and video cameras—remains homogenous across the entire sample.

The Importance of Digital Quality and Indifference of Device Design and Accessories

Quite often, the choice of a purchased smartphone was dictated by the param-eters of its camera participants would use to film their exercises. They put a special emphasis on the quality of the pictures taken, paying a particular attention to the resolution they required, the matrix, etc., as well as available recording functions (acceleration, time-lapse). The recorded material was required to record even minute details and in HD quality so that it could be used for online publications.

The design of the device was judged as completely irrelevant—in fact, only one person perceived the appearance of a smartphone as significant while the construction of the camera and the possibility of filming from different perspectives (front and rear cameras) was often highlighted.

Some respondents emphasized the necessity to protect their smartphones from damage by using waterproof or dustproof covers, but in most cases protection was of little importance and in some cases (it was substituted by ordinary plastic bags during rowing).

The marginalization of smartphones accessories is noteworthy as it signifi-cantly contrasts with their great importance during running or gym workouts. The respondents repeatedly recalled numerous accessories accompanying their activities: filming drones (horse riding, parkour), special tripods and fixings, e.g., mounting cameras on a mirror (ballroom dance, pole dance) or one's chest (western-style horse riding). However, they were not used very often, apart from mountain biking, by fixing a camera to the handlebars; paragliding—fastening to the harness; classic horse riding—fixing to the helmet; and pole dance—a tripod. Observation of workouts indicates an absolute lack of professionalization of the filming activity itself, which mainly results from the lack of proper accessories. Quite often, smartphones are set in haphazard places and propped by random objects found in the immediate environment of users (mattresses, training equipment, dance hall equipment, etc.):

"(. . .) This is going to sound weird, but I had my [smartphone] resting on a shoe somehow or on a concrete column that was there. Or I had it resting on my bag . . . that I always carry with me and put aside" (female figure rollerblader);

"There are those yoga blocks at the gym—we put them together, rest a phone against them; various practical things, or we put them on the backpack. No special things . . ." (female ballroom dancer).

The process of self-recording gives the impression of being completely makeshift, unplanned, and haphazard. This results in time wasted on search for the right arrangement to achieve the desired perspective and quality, which lengthens the training sessions and affects their course.[13]

The contrast between the required high quality digital recording and the lack of the use of appropriate, relatively inexpensive equipment, which would increase that quality and facilitate the recording process, may result from several factors. Amateurs and paraprofessionals do not have adequate knowledge and/or professional support, e.g., training staff that professionals have at their disposal. In the cohort, only three individuals regularly use the assistance of a trainer (except one participant engaging with a trainer remotely), and most consider it unnecessary. The respondents feel that they are self-sufficient.[14] Restricted to their own resources, they "cope" with home-made methods both in the planning and implementation of training sessions, and in the use of media technologies during those training activities. In addition, it is very likely that their sporting activity (and the accompanying publishing activity) does not require great quality, both in terms of the achieved sports results or media materials, to reach for highly specialist accessories, including other cameras than those built into the smartphone.

Their amateur or paraprofessional approach to sport goes hand-in-hand with the same approach to using media technologies, namely video recording, in exercises. On the other hand, one could say that if it were not for the use of commonly available cameras, users' ability to achieve and stimulate progress would be significantly reduced, as most of them engage in sports on their own and do not use professional support. They point out unanimously that, due to accessibility of other individuals' video materials and the possibility of video recording of their own workouts, they can reach their goals alone.

Ambivalent Nature of Media Technologies

While video recording is often an indispensable element of training to respondents practicing niche disciplines, the camera is not always seen as most important technology. In many cases, it becomes an "invisible" and obvious technology, particularly for respondents who watch the material mainly or only after the training is completed. The camera tracks their activity, but at some point they stop noticing its presence ("I forget about the camera during the flight . . ."). Thus, training takes place regardless of its presence, although there may be incidental moments when the device is noticed. This happens mainly when the workout does not go according to plan, when unexpected problems appear which prompt users to consider stopping recording their performance ("If I get mad . . . I prefer that nobody watches and records it, I prefer to avoid such situations"). All in all, however, the majority of respondents (nine individuals) who engage in amateur sports, do use a camera to watch the recordings after finishing a workout.

In many situations, however, the camera is at the core of their interest and the subject of fundamental interaction during the workout. Not only does it structure a workout, but also transforms it. Thus, not only the camera is constantly noticed and repeatedly engaged with during a workout, but the recording becomes the end-goal of the physical activity, and can even serve as its necessary condition.[15]

Conversely, situations when the camera is deliberately absent and its use entirely eliminated from a training session can be observed, too. In such cases, the goal is a "detox," a resignation from the use of technology aimed at sole commitment to training, leading to incidental desaturation.[16] As the video camera becomes more ubiquitous, its presence can lead to additional pressure felt by the training individuals, prompting them to abandon the device. The research shows, however, that only amateurs can afford to opt out from video recording.

While some of the aforementioned technologies are seen as "invisible," other devices, including the timer on the training room wall, the paraglider variograph, the onboard computer on the bike, are completely "untransparent." Exercising individuals reach for them, look at them, and interact with them throughout the training session. These technologies clearly structure the training: i.e., they divide it into stages, sequences, and cycles; in other words, they determine the manner, direction, and pace of movement.

In certain cases, the specific "visibility" and "invisibility" of some technologies can be of a situational character. For example, a smartphone with a launched Endomondo application tucked into its user's pocket does not generate constant awareness of it operating; when taken out to snap a picture, however, it becomes visible and the awareness of its presence and use returns. There are also technologies of which individuals are practically not aware during a workout, such as GPS embedded in tracking applications, e.g., used by skiers.

In summary, individuals display diverse levels of awareness of the presence and visibility of technologies and the video camera seems to be particularly susceptible to that perception change. It can be positioned in an "invisible" and easy to forget about place (e.g., on a helmet), but it may equally well become the center of its user's attention. This, in turn, determines the scope and the potential implications of its use.

PROCESSUAL SATURATION

Processes Mediated via Video Recording Technologies

The use of a video camera by niche disciplines' enthusiasts appear to mediate three main processes: analysis, commemoration, and communication.

Analysis

The camera used during exercise records the image and allows users to follow and examine their own activity (movements, ambient conditions, equipment operation) either during or after the workout. Retrospective reception dominates, but five respondents (all paraprofessionals) use the option of receiving the recorded video during their training.

Due to the specificity of physical activity (changes in movement, body position, etc.) self-recording is used for three main reasons. First of all, it records often undetected changes in movement or position (in the mirror, or even by an observer), due to the highly dynamic nature of activity. Subsequently, due to the acceleration and deceleration function, it allows for the viewing of details which are usually difficult to detect with the naked eye. Lastly, due the location of the camera at a certain distance and angle, one can obtain a side view, mimicking the perspective of another person, which can be important in assessing the overall effect of an activity:

"... course it's easier with a camera. When we look at the mirror we dance a bit more slowly and take notice of all the mistakes. But there are certain figures when we can't look at the mirror as we're also doing acrobatics. I'm upside down, facing my partner's back. No way you can have a peek. Without this option, or the mirror, or the camera we'd have to do the figures alone and correct each other. That'd be difficult cause it's impossible to check acrobatics this way" (female ballroom dancer).

Therefore, one of the biggest triggers for the implementation of further video recording functions, such as error analysis, is the desire of users to see themselves from a particular perspective. Most of them declare the need to see their performance from the side, how they look, and what their activity looks like in the context of their surroundings. They want to see themselves, but not in the mirror or through the eyes of others, but on the screen. They want to gain the opportunity to look at themselves in the mediated material. This particular curiosity brings on further functions that are fulfilled by video recording.

The basic goal of the reception, both retrospective and simultaneous, is to eliminate errors on different levels:

- firstly: increase the awareness of mistakes made,
- secondly: capture them and analyze (sometimes in slow motion) a given fragment of the training, followed by a comprehensive, critical evaluation of its course in order to determine the causes of those errors and determine possible solutions,
- thirdly: correction (including: re-recording of the same element).

When watching the recordings post factum, conclusions are drawn for the next training sessions, for example, a cyclist returns to the completed route and corrects the errors they identified while playing the footage or a western-style rider adjusts their sitting position. Similar behavior was declared in the context of paragliding, skiing, rowing, classic riding, MMA, and figure roller-blading:

"The video shows that I *am* [emphasis added] tossing about. It's not smooth. This shows me what mistakes I'm making" (male paraglider);

"I don't know why it [sometimes] goes wrong. Then I film myself and it's all clear: the arm's too high or something like that. It's a tiny detail that I normally don't see. It's only when I see the video I can correct something and make it OK. So that's what I normally do—I correct the mistakes I see on the video. And then everything's alright" (female pole dancer);

"When I do the snatch I let go slowly and then I see where I made a mistake and where I didn't" (male cross-fitter);

"(. . .) then I check if I go evenly when I jump over some obstacles, some bars . . . was the horse's head in the right position; it's the same with my arms 'cause I tend to look down on the horse when I shouldn't" (female classic horse rider);

"(. . .) I can see what mistakes I made, e.g., put my arm wrong. I walked too slowly. Minor details you can't see while lying on the mat, that can only be seen when you see yourself from a distance" (male MMA).

In one case, the recorded material was used to consult a trainer remotely (cross-fit).

While self-recording sometimes turns out to be insufficient or too poor, generally the possibility of catching errors is seen as enhanced when the person is additionally filmed by a third party.

"If I mount the camera on the bike or the helmet (. . .) on the crossbar, I film the whole route, i.e., the way I ride. This captures all the mistakes I make, too. Now, if we ride in groups . . . and someone's got a camera—that's even better. Not only am I able to spot technical mistakes I make while riding but I can also analyze myself, the very way I act . . ., my legwork, posture, is it just the wheel, the rear wheel, what goes on in the front or the back, or on the side" (male mountain biker).

Video recording aiming at the elimination of errors in real time transforms the workout into repetitive, schematic cycles. Depending on whether the training person uses someone else's video tutorial or not, it can be done in two ways:

"We put the phone up. We start recording, we record with or without music—depends what we need. Then we play the video and check whether we did the figure the way we had imagined. Does it look the same? Does it look good? Did we make a mistake we hadn't known of before? Often when you do a figure, the body doesn't feel it's making a mistake, you can only notice it when you look at it from a distance. We then do some checking and correcting and record again. And we repeat until we get it right" (female ballroom dancer).

exercise recorded → video playback/drawing conclusions → repeated exercise recorded

watching of a video tutorial → exercise recorded → video playback/drawing conclusions → watching of a video tutorial → repeated exercise recorded

Figure 4.1.   Two dominant cycles of video recording during a workout.
Source: own elaboration.

Such cycles become increasingly automated, and sometimes modified, for example, with the crowning element in the form of editing and then publishing of the recorded material on social media platforms:

"(. . .) suppose I'm taking a photo of myself. I make another series. During the break I do some photoshopping. During the next one I post it" (male fitness bodybuilder).

The analysis is usually focused on details, small aspects, such as elements that cannot be noticed, for example, in the mirror. There is an assumption that the video camera sees more than a human being, both the exercising person and the third party watching them. The opinions of other observers are actually often contested:

"(. . .) my friends started to tell me: make a video of what you do to see what mistakes you're making. Because we keep telling you but you can't see it. When you see it on video, you'll realize the mistakes. Then I go, oh, yeah, I'm not straightening my leg properly or I'm not raising my arm high enough. What I'm saying is, when someone told me about my mistakes I couldn't quite picture it until I saw them with my own eyes" (female traceur).

Due to its functions (repeated playback, deceleration, acceleration), the video camera can capture the core of the problem. The perfecting takes place immediately; not on the occasion of the next training session with the aim of avoiding duplication of errors and stimulating faster progress:

"This must be quickly corrected before your muscular memory notices it or memorizes the wrong figure as the right one. . . . You've got to know these things and act straight away" (male calisthenics practitioner).

Exercise and filming become integrated activities and a particular symbiosis takes place. Based on the analysis of the recording, the movements are performed more accurately and often in a more attractive manner. As a result, the person exercising appreciates the effects, which in some cases is more important than the praise from a potential trainer.[17] In disciplines where aesthetics counts (e.g., pole dance, ballroom dance, figure roller-blading), the respondents repeatedly emphasized the importance of the so-called side view. It is a rather striking consideration, taking into account an impression made on a potential viewer; an impression concerning not only correctness, but also attractiveness. In addition, a positive result of the recording self-assessment increases its chance of being published on social media.[18]

On the other hand, there are some drawbacks resulting from the process of watching recordings while training. Usually, reviewing of the recorded material is perceived as a time dedicated to relaxation. It is a moment of rest between a series of exercises, but also the time of loosened focus from one's body. It results in participants assuming casual positions (hunching, leaning against objects, or bending their bodies) while watching the footage from their workouts, which is contradictive to what they had been working on a moment earlier. They stare at the smartphone screen, taking anywhere from mere seconds to entire minutes, while perpetuating inappropriate body positions at times lasting relatively long. Training transforms into alternate sequences of physical exercise and passivity, with the latter becoming the time of media activity. There is a temporary suspension of either the movement or the reception of the media content.

Visual analysis applies not only to one's own mistakes, but also to the surroundings, which can affect a workout. This applies in particular to disciplines in which specific external conditions (the weather, the landform) and relevant adaptation to them can help achieve better sports effects in disciplines such as mountain biking, paragliding, skiing, rowing, and classic horse riding. One of such conditions is cooperation with others in team sports (rowing), disciplines involving animals (classic horse-riding, western style horse-riding) or sports often practiced in larger groups (skiing, mountain biking, paragliding, ballroom dancing). Footage recording in this context has also a motivational meaning:

"It was cool when after practice you could pick out who slows us down or speeds us up or what needs correcting (. . .). When you don't have the video camera you might ignore it or pull a little less" (female rower);

"(. . .) of course I straighten myself. I don't hunch. You do the pose differently because you know this is going to be on film. The riders' world is very hermetic and I know it's gonna get back to me, that I'm not sitting straight or I'm pulling the horse. . . . I'm more involved because I want a record of doing my best" (female classic horse rider).

Apart from the elimination of errors and maximizing training possibilities, self-recording analysis is aimed at memorizing movements, positions, and figures. This applies above all to the disciplines involving the creation of one own's sequences or choreography, i.e., ballroom dance, pole dance, parkour, and calisthenics. The performed elements are reproduced many times and thus repeatedly recorded and played, which helps to memorize them:

"I'm doing a combo, a combination of a few figures. I'm not able to memorize it so I have to record it to be able to go back to it later" (female pole dancer).

It is worth emphasizing that a video recording analysis usually starts at a particular stage of the exercising person's development in a given sport discipline. Sometimes the beginnings are recorded, but not so much for the purpose of errors analysis, remembering or maximizing effects, but to memorialize them. However, the pursuit of a higher advancement with the use of a video camera in training reveals itself over time. This is particularly important for paraprofessionals whose work is linked to a sporting activity. It also becomes helpful for advanced amateurs who want to continue developing. In most cases, however, it is undesirable at the initial stage. It could discourage the exercising person from a particular form of activity due to the dissatisfaction with oneself caused by a disheartening number of errors or slow progress:

"(. . .) I was really scared to record myself (. . .). Well, I'm not very flexible, I mean, I wasn't, at least at the very beginning (. . .). I already knew what it looked like. I didn't want to record it but with time (. . .). I guess it wouldn't make much sense for me to run around with a camera while learning something new" (female traceur);

"(. . .) more difficult elements—because I can already do the basic stuff like crossovers or backward rollerblading, so this doesn't need observing to learn. But when I'm doing more advanced elements I rewind the film a couple of times or I slow it down to watch this particular moment and see how it works out and what it looks like technically" (female figure rollerblader).

A video camera does not serve as a tool for initial education, but for improvement, and, more precisely, for self-improvement. It seems to expose errors and to strip away the illusion of perfection. It finds use in training when there is a desire to enhance efficiency in the pursuit of a particular goal. At more advanced stages, it also addresses the desire to memorialize particular stages of development. It is possible, among other things, due to the use of a video camera as it allows the exercising person to see what normally they wouldn't see. It allows one to visualize as well as analyze errors, and given the lack of trainers or training partners in most of the studied cases, the camera is an essential tool for self-sufficiency, or at least, it facilitates such an illusion. By assisting self-diagnosis followed by self-correction, it allows to reach further stages of development without a professional support (trainer, instructor). It also, however, generates the risk of ignorance leading to imperceptibility of some errors, which can potentially to hinder one's own development. Relying on oneself, on a video camera, and possibly other technological aids may not be universally sufficient for continuous development. For an amateur or paraprofessional sportsperson, however, it can be a satisfactory and rewarding level, potentially much higher than when engaging in sports without said media technologies. It is particularly noteworthy that the individuals determine the satisfactory level of achievement based on the recording, however, they seem to be aware of the limitations resulting from this form of self-perfection:

"(. . .) I don't know if I can achieve some kind of super high level, I mean—it definitely is some level. . . I think. But it's not like I feel pressure to reach some level of those evolutions. I simply try to shape it up to make it better and better" (female figure rollerblader);

"(. . .) I can learn the snatch by myself. If you're clever enough, you'll do it. I know I won't reach perfection—that's not possible. But for the sake of your own [progress], I think you can do it" (male cross-fitter).

Memorializing

The second purpose of using the camera is to memorialize the workouts. On the one hand, it serves as simple archiving of training notes, allowing one to reach for some solutions, ideas, results, etc., in the future. On the other hand, it is a systematic documentation of the path of one's own development, enabling progress evaluation in a short and long-term dimension. Western-style horse riding, based on close cooperation between horse and rider, brings effects in a longer perspective and only after a substantial period of time it's possible to see one's own or their animal's progress. Due to the relationship that is built (with other individuals as well as animals), such materials become sentimental tokens:

"(. . .) when I've got it on my hard drive, I go back to it and it's really nice, too. Those are my memories, after all. Each video even if it's boring to normal viewers—I mean, how many times can you watch a horse's head and whatever's going on around it—for me those are memories. Here I suddenly remember something that happened. Here a deer jumped onto the road in front of me. . . . A nice short piece, when I come back to it, I watch it. Yeah, the weather was really great. It was such a pleasant ride. The horse was obedient. It did what I wanted it to do. I didn't have a hard time with him, or anything like that. It's great to keep those memories, because they're—you know—simply pleasant" (female classic horse rider).

Also in other disciplines new skills are acquired over time, and when individuals see their own progress, they want to immortalize it. In particular, when they reach some exceptional achievements, they want to preserve them for the future. In such cases, when those achievements bear the quality of uniqueness (like a jump in parkour), memorializing them becomes extremely important:

"If I do something really big then I record it. . . . The more you practice the more you can do with your body. It's something that takes really hard work, many years of hard work—if there's a jump that's big, massive and heavy, say technically . . . It's not like we do this every day. Our daily practice is usually sitting on one wall and doing 100 push-ups, 100 crunches, 100 sit-ups, till your muscles quit. But these great jumps you can see on our videos are like the fruit of our workouts (. . .). That's why we want to film it the best way possible" (female traceur).

A video featuring a high achievement or performance serves as a summary of the current path of development and is often the subject of publication on the web, which gains new functions for both authors and recipients as well as the broadly defined sport discipline.

The individuals return to recordings of their training sessions after a while as those hold a sentimental value for them. Participants observe their progress, but also nostalgically reminisce, sometimes in a company of other exercising partners (rowing, skiing, paragliding), and thus, the watching acquires social values. Memories trigger vivid emotions, motivation to continue physical activity, and they stimulate the desire to take on even greater challenges. Mementos in the form of videos become also a source of relaxation and detachment from reality, especially when a given form of activity cannot be performed at a particular time. Some of these materials end up on the web (mainly on YouTube) and are the subject of sharing a passion with both familiar and anonymous recipients.

Communication

Communicating about physical activity is the third goal of recording exercises on video. The footage created during one's own training or its culmination in the form of competitions, achievements, shows, etc., after meeting certain requirements, is published on social media platforms. Most respondents (eleven) post such content, with eight individuals on a regular basis, compared to three who do that only sporadically. Some of the materials are made available to a limited audience (trainers, friends from the same discipline), others become publicly available. Regardless of their reach, they serve two main functions: self-presentation and promotion.

Self-presentation and Promotion

Photos and videos depicting physical activity posted via Facebook, Instagram, Snapchat, or YouTube are used for self-presentation. The exact nature of those posts, however, differs depending whether they were published by amateurs, or paraprofessionals, with the latter placing emphasis on the marketing and promotional attributes. The researched amateurs do not hide they boastful intentions ("Oh! Look, I'm working out!" female pole dancer) that they publish for "likes," comments, and jealousy of others. For some, the mere fact of regular activity is already a source of pride; for others, it lies in steady progress, achievements, or record setting.

Regardless of their nature, all posts are a source of satisfaction with the achieved sports effects, but also their visual representation:

"I usually do those things [i.e., publish films] for myself. Unless there's something I do well, then I can share it" (female western-style horse rider);

"When I'm filming something and decide: 'Wow, this is good!' then I can show it off. Then nothing can stop me from making a video and posting it on Instagram or YouTube. But if I've got something 'smaller' or something I just want to show to my friends, then I post it on Facebook. I've got the privacy setting on so someone who doesn't know me, can't view my profile" (female traceur);

"We never post our rehearsal videos because they never look the way they should. We only post show videos in full gear or from workshops. All top notch" (female ballroom dancer).

Self-presentation concerns not only showing oneself as an athletic, active, visually attractive person, but also the emotions experienced during physical activity. Participants who publish content strive to present to others their self-satisfaction, overcoming adversity, their achievements, or the joy derived from exercises related either to working on their own body or staying in a particular environment, e.g., weather or landscape conditions:

"(. . .) well, you sometimes want to share what you do, or the effects of what you do, with others. All sorts of cameras were available earlier but they did not give justice to how you feel riding a bike or going on an expedition, or being in a rough mountainous terrain and you want to show off your achievements. With a video camera I can bring the viewer closer to what I felt, more or less, while doing some acrobatics on my bike, or braving difficult terrain or visiting some area that is not accessible to most ordinary people" (male mountain biker);

"It brings me joy to know that I overcame a weakness, I broke some boundaries and I just want to show it to others so that they can enjoy it with me" (female rower).

While amateurs film and publish voluntarily and rather more willingly, paraprofessionals feel the pressure and weariness. To them, self-presentation means the promotion of themselves and the business they run. Paraprofessionals do not limit themselves to simply recording a workout and publishing it on the web sometime afterward. They process and publish recordings by themselves, often even during training sessions, which distinguishes them from amateurs. Also, they demonstrate great proficiency in the knowledge and skills of operating graphic and editing applications:

"It would be too boring to watch if I posted it on social media. Left leg, right leg. . ., that's why you accelerate it. I've got a thirty-second long video [whereas in fact] it's five-seconds long. It's a gif thing, one-two, one-two. Cool. You can slow it down, too. Let's say we're dealing with a really quick figure but someone wants to see how it looks technically—where the elbows are, whatever. You can slow it down, too. There are different motives for photos, some distortions. And so on, and so forth" (male calisthenics practitioner).

Paraprofessionals publish regularly and across a variety of platforms. Physical activity is integrated not only with filming, photography, and processing, but also with intense reflection about where and how to communicate the content best. These processes are intertwined, but they do not create a sense of satisfaction, as it was in the case of amateurs, but fatigue and weariness. The pressure to publish triggers a sense of resistance, followed by frustration:

"I'm fine with it now, but at the beginning I had those huge qualms about doing it" (male cross-fitter);

"(. . .) it used to be more condensed, the only thing you focused on was the practice, now you have to worry a little . . ., it's not only passion anymore but also work . . . Sometimes you go to work out and you have a bad day. You don't feel like taking any photos. You just want to do this workout, go home and go to bed. That's all. . . But you need to mind the business. I have to do something. I have to post a photo because I haven't posted one in, say, two days. . . When I didn't have my fanpage I didn't even need to take my phone to a workout. You know, it used to disturb me, distract me. Someone calling, someone texting. The breaks were always longer than they were supposed to be. It just didn't work the way it should 100 percent . . . I've been working out for a really long time now and I don't need it for myself, to look at it later. I need it more for work, to earn money. That's why I'm promoting myself" (male fitness body builder);

"[Because I am a horse rider] I get offers from, e.g., sports clothing companies. You know, I do feel kind of pressure to do more, to show more. . . . At the beginning it was some kind of fun . . . but when I opened an account [to public], it turned out that it may help you gain a tiny bit of popularity" (female classic horse rider).

Paraprofessionals achieve the promotional effect due to self-presentation, mainly of their appearance, course of activity, and sports achievements that make them credible in the eyes of potential customers or advertisers. They also use publications for motivational purposes (e.g., in the form of feedback from others[19]) and competitions (through comparison with rivals). However, the primary goal is marketing and published films as well as photos to promote both the individuals and their level of advancement. Thus, paraprofessionals focus on their commercial activities with a strong emphasis on marketing. In addition to self-presentation, amateurs also declare the promotion of broadly defined physical activity and their niche discipline, which particularly applies to emerging disciplines.[20]

AESTHETICIZATION AND DEAESTHETICIZATION

Publishing on social media platforms mainly pertains to Facebook, Instagram, and YouTube with a few participants using Snapchat. Each of those media platforms sets out a specific framework for posts, including written and unwritten technical and socio-cultural rules that define the features of the published content. In addition and on an individual level, these platforms perform slightly different functions. Amateur respondents declare that they perceive Facebook as a nonpublic communication tool, i.e., limited to a defined group, but to paraprofessionals it is the main promotion platform. Instagram, on the other hand, is seen as the main platform gathering individuals who share a particular passion: it is therefore the main source of access and the platform for publishing visual materials about niche sports both for amateurs and paraprofessionals. Similarly, YouTube serves as a valuable source of knowledge. However, it is rarely used for publishing by amateurs and more often by paraprofessionals. Snapchat, overall is used in few cases, but it is becoming more popular for promotional (paraprofessionals) and self-presentation (amateurs) purposes.

Publishing photos and videos pertaining to physical activity on those three main social media platforms is chiefly characterized by the aesthetic appeal in both technical and visual dimensions. The technical aestheticization lies in the strive to achieve the highest technical quality of a photo or film which requires the use of a video camera that records movies with a certain quality, but also the potential technical processing that enhances its visual aspects:

"If this [recording] is for me only and I need to view it, it doesn't [have to be in high quality], but if I had to make a more important film I wouldn't do it with this video camera [phone camera]" (female pole dancer);

"I've purged my Instagram account completely and I'm starting anew because I shot my films with some kind of 'toaster' and I thought, 'we have a good camera, let's do it with something solid and post good quality videos'" (female traceur);

"I upload it to my smartphone Photoshop. It takes 10 seconds to adjust sharp-
ness, adjust this white balance thing, to make it a tad better. Often, when the
light is too sharp, the photo is overexposed. For instance, when I'm taking photos at the workout, the top of the photo [on my shoulders] is badly overexposed,
you can't see various details, so you need to turn down this lighting to make
it darker. Then it starts to look better and you can post it to your fanpage right
away. It takes five, ten minutes" (male fitness body builder).

Sometimes striving for a certain technical level requires "circumventing" the
technical capabilities of the application, for example by using special applications to change to the film format suitable for Instagram. Users find remedies
for the imperfections of the medium, and accomplish their publication goals
by exploiting the features of a given platform:

"Videos in the 1:1 format simply look worse. Instagram has already changed
it, now you can choose 16:9 for example, but earlier you had to resort to using
other programs, which added those white or black stripes at the top of the video,
which made it meet the Instagram requirements" (male fitness body builder).

The respondents focus on the technical aesthetics to achieve a clean, non-
blurry image and appropriate brightness when lighting is insufficient. For
many, this is also important when they recorded videos only for themselves.[21]
In any case, the pursuit of appropriate self-presentation and promotion of
physical activity determines the use of appropriate equipment (digital camera) and software (processing and editing applications). Additionally, and due
to the importance of its numerous detail occurring simultaneously, physical
activity enforces the use of specialist technology so that the resulting material
meets the expectations of both the exercising individuals and the potential
recipients. Technical quality of the material must be matched by the quality
of the exercise performance or workout, although the latter is relative and
determined by the exercising person. Sometimes participants experience
anxiety and fear that the recording quality will be insufficient or that technical
problems will occur at the most precious moment:

"(. . .) sometimes someone does something brilliant but the camera switches off
by itself. And the second, third or fourth time is not so brilliant anymore. . . . I
don't know if I can do it tomorrow again and I'd like to film the best version of
it. . . . It's really important to us that the recording quality should reflect all the
effort we put in it" (female traceur).

The second dimension of the aesthetization of photographic and video content concerns the visual qualities of the content of the produced material
and its mechanism is converse to technical aesthetics. It is not the physical

activity that determines the application of a particular technology, but it is the technology that affects specific contexts and elements of physical activity. Aiming to create a film or a photograph with particular qualities requires certain conditions to be met by the location of training and the appearance of the exercising person as well as their surroundings. Facebook, Instagram, and YouTube are platforms which "demand" material that is "nice" and generates interest. The appearance of the exercising person and the specificity of the surroundings must meet special requirements. There is pressure and the expectation of meeting the requirement of sufficient attractiveness levels. However, the respondents indicate that naturalness, realism, and accessibility of content is also strongly required:

"If I have beautiful surroundings—the way I like it, i.e., sunshine on a bridge with water flowing underneath. . . and beautiful greenery around, then [I record it]. And if needed, I add a little commentary too" (female rower);

"Now it's completely different. Now people wear trendy clothes to the gym, nice clothes, so that they look tasteful. . . . Before, nobody even thought about taking a photo of themselves. . . . Now, let's say we have this trend. . .—you can tell that they [the photos] are taken as if off guard; just during workout. [Such photos] are even more popular than the posed ones. It's because people like seeing this naturalness; the way it really looks. . . and it's those pictures, hand-held shots (the so-called selfies) that are better received" (male fitness body builder).

Overall, the previously analyzed requirement of an appropriate advancement level or progress in sport is additionally supplemented by the requirement that the content of the material must be aesthetic to qualify for publishing. The synergy of the sports level and the aesthetic degree of the produced materials is once again evident. However, with the emergence of a new communication platform, Snapchat, the users have adapted to its new aesthetic standards, which are characterized by the lack of visual perfection, facilitating therefore a kind of deaestheticization.

Snapchat shows fleeting moments from everyday life and the published materials are quite ephemeral, less polished, and ordinary, hence, often imperfect. It also forces frequent updating of the profile since the number of viewers depends on the frequency of publishing. This generates even greater traffic, but also different aesthetics, both on a technical and visual level. Due to the mechanisms governing social media platforms, the content becomes less training-oriented and more focused on the broadly defined sport:

"Let's say I'm going to work out with a friend. We do some exercises and I gladly record them. When I get back from my workout. . . something to do with my business that is not directly related to sports, more indirectly—I try to post it, share it and record it" (male body builder).

With time, the necessity to constantly adapt to the requirements of the medium, however, becomes a burden and it can be compared to the aforementioned pressure on paraprofessionals to publish often and a lot. Discomfort generated by that affects amateurs as well. It results, among other outcomes, from the video camera's excessive impact on the course of training, pressure of competition, or even health deterioration:[22]

> "I've noticed that the more individuals record themselves the more they try to practice for the camera. That's why I like to have a no-camera workout sometimes. No camera, no thinking about what to do, what to record. . . . This week nothing. I practice for myself only. And I don't care if it looks ok or not" (female traceur).

Prolonged pressure leading to forced training for the camera gives rise to the need to abandon it. Desaturation in the context of video recording of selected training sessions is, however, a rarely declared outcome.

FUNCTIONS, GAINS, AND LOSSES OF VIDEO RECORDING

Consequently, it can be said that video recording fulfills several basic functions, both at the level of playing the content and its publication. In the former case, the implementation of these processes serves self-improvement by addressing errors, maximizing opportunities, and speeding up the process of memorizing. In the latter, it consolidates and commemorates the training process and progress achieved for the future. In both cases, this allows for achieving a relative level of self-sufficiency in training and self-satisfaction with one's own achievements.

Functions and Meta-functions

The publishing of the created films reveals their subsequent functions. They constitute a tool for self-presentation and promotion of the exercising individuals themselves, their activities, as well as the sport discipline they practice, and broadly understood physical activity. As a subject of popular circulation on the Internet, the published videos begin to play meta-functions by becoming a source of knowledge for others. As some of the respondents reported, it was actually the watching of a video material on the web that triggered their interest in a new sport discipline. Watching the materials published mainly on YouTube serves as the initiation and the moment of instilling interest in the discipline. Later stages of engagement with YouTube and Instagram provides a "wealth of knowledge" that prompts respondents' development. It's aided by instructors (e.g., skiing techniques), tutorials (e.g., how to enter a pole dance figure), motivational films and inspirational materials encouraging to try new solutions and create one's own (e.g., combining styles in ballroom dance). Publicly available films inspire the practitioners to not cease in their efforts and set goals to which they want to aspire. Respondents also become, in their own opinion, self-sufficient,[23] and even ready to teach others:

"Having someone else's videos, their "progress" to look at, all the basic workshops and what have you. . . I'm able to reach the same place they have reached, all I need is the Internet. . . . Having the Internet and being eager. . . having all the tools, I'm simply able to achieve anything in calisthenics" (male calisthenics practitioner).

By uploading their own video materials, respondents contribute to the knowledge and inspiration of other individuals. In addition, they promote an active lifestyle and popularize the discipline they practice. Above all, they take part in its evolution. The impact of social media videos on the transformation of disciplines is one of the most important dimensions of the mediatization of physical activity. Those who exercise publish films presenting new training methods and thus, depending on the discipline, new techniques or styles of movement, as well as illustrating changes in the rules and rules of conduct in given sport disciplines. As they explain, due to the general access to such materials, the changes can be very quickly implemented by others and propagated by them in the form of subsequent videos:

"If someone comes up with a new exercise and makes it popular, they usually do it by posting a video online. That's how it works. . . . I've recently seen . . . a really cool exercise. . . . You do it on two barbells which are, like, on one side. They're stuck in a kind of a stand on two sides. They have plates attached to them. You can use it to do flies and go down to the middle. . . This exercise has become popular because some bodybuilder or fitness guy posted a video online. I don't think it would have reached me here in Wrocław all the way from the States just by word of mouth" (male fitness body builder);

"Bachata used to have a Dominican character. It wasn't until it became more recognizable online and individuals started to watch those videos. . . they were able to get through to other styles such as zooka, samba or salsa. Now some elements of one dance are being incorporated into another. It gets mixed all the time to make it as interesting as possible" (female ballroom dancer);

"There's this girl who shows her practice videos in which she shows those really interesting and diverse bar arrangements that the horse goes over. . . . It's
not merely three or four bars as it's usually done at a normal practice, those are
proper arrangements. Those are circles, loops. . . . It certainly is a form of learning, I've used it quite a few times" (female classic horse rider).

Certainly, some disciplines, especially emerging ones, are more susceptible to
rapid changes and dynamic development while others, more well-established,
less so. Therefore, the nature of the discipline determines the volume of
change introduced by practitioners striving to achieve better results. In pole
dance and parkour, new figures and positions are proposed by amateurs:

"(. . .) spread really quickly. An amateur does something new and in a week's
time everyone will be doing the same move because they saw it on the Internet.
[Parkour] is a different kind of sport and it's difficult to come up with new
moves to inspire people, to make them try to copy it or to come up with something totally new. But it is also important. . . because people get inspired all the
time. With a new style, they find out what can improve the way they practice"
(female traceur).[24]

In addition to the evolution of techniques, styles, and thus entire disciplines,
significant changes in practitioners' behavior, generally accepted rules in the
discipline, and the speed at which they are introduced can be observed. It is
particularly noticeable in the activities involving animals:

"[YouTube has huge impact on western style horse riding] because it is still not
a very popular sport in Poland. It's been here for about 15 years and it keeps
developing. Every now and then there's a new method coming out. . . . In the
last five years [the discipline] has changed dramatically in terms of the riding
style. At the beginning individuals. . . used to sit far in front of the horse. Then it
changed—they moved more to the back. Now it's changed again and they have
to sit in the middle. . . . With those changes, there's a huge gap between what
was then and what is now. . . . [If it wasn't for the Internet, the changes would
have taken place] very slowly. It would take years for the books to be published,
for the changes to reach us" (female western style horse rider).

Only occasionally, the respondents pay attention to the risks associated with
the publication, watching, and modeling on the videos of other amateurs or
paraprofessionals, and thus potential effects of errors, including dangers and
accidents. In principle, the problem of the reliability of sources hardly ever
appears in the respondents' statements. The risk of relying on amateur materials while engaging in independent training without the assistance of a specialist is generally not recognized. However, they are aware of other hazards
resulting from self-recording.

Gains and Losses

Some of the losses and gains from video recording differ for individual respondents. However, universally recognized losses arising from self-recording include time-wasting before, during, and after training. This results from the need to prepare for filming, pausing, and watching, which significantly prolong the training. In addition, a considerable amount of time is devoted to watching the videos after training:

> "(. . .) those technologies, as smartphones themselves, bother me more than help me because they make my practice longer. . . with making videos and taking photos the training takes longer than it would without it" (female rower).

Pressure is another element resulting in significant losses. For paraprofessionals, it stems from the necessity to film for promotional purposes. A workout determined by recording is based on other forms of or the level of involvement in physical activity. To a lesser extent, its goals are of an internal nature since most often they are triggered by external environment and thus are socially-oriented. Pressure can sometimes result from a specific video of a competing user and is often triggered by comparison to others who practice the same discipline and publish their achievements online. This leads to the loss of pleasure in training and in some cases also has a negative impact on health (i.e., the aforementioned example of practicing pole dance while using only one side of the body). Respondents report that engaging in exercise in front of the video camera sometimes results in tension, which disappears when the recording is stopped and individuals can change position of their body and relax. They fill the time watching the recording just made. The screen of the video camera or a smartphone sometimes facilitates an "escape" from subsequent attempts, especially when one experiences weariness or fatigue.

The nature of video recording can be paradoxical at times. On the one hand, filming allows the exercising person to focus on training, on the effects, and on details. On the other hand, however, the respondents report it makes it difficult to focus. First of all, the workout is often interrupted. Secondly, the focus on recording leads to the omission of other elements, especially in the surrounding environment. In consequence, regular use of the video camera may trigger to "detox" from recording, isolation, which sometimes poses a challenge itself and requires self-discipline to give it up.

The main benefits include the effects of visualization of one's own physical activity. Firstly, one gains the opportunity to see oneself, to get a side view from the perspective of a third person that is often absent during the workout. Sometimes it is accompanied by the possibility to observe the surroundings of the exercise location and drawing useful conclusions. Also, the visualization of the activity can lead to self-acceptance, self-satisfaction, or identification of mistakes that can be addressed. The recording reveals elements not visible to the naked eye during an activity and those can be discovered only via recording from a different perspective, resulting in subsequent attempts to correct any identified errors. Also, greater control over the course of the training is achieved and memorizing movements is made easier.

In the long-term, video recording gives exercising individuals the opportunity to compare and view their own progress over time. It allows them to build their own story, and thus becomes a kind of a sentimental keepsake. For para-professionals, it is the main tool for promoting themselves and the source of their income, while for amateurs, it can serve as a self-presentation tool, garnering social approval, reinforcement and motivation to continue their efforts.

Self-improvement and Co-improvement

It is mainly the perception of benefits—and not losses—that leads to basic mediatization mechanisms occurrence, and it does so on a very large scale. It results from the saturation of physical activity with the recording and watching processes, which are become increasingly intertwined. The mediatization mechanism is based on the visual mapping of physical activity, its publication and subsequent watching, which are interrelated and repetitive. This tendency is revealed both at the micro level of exercising individuals' action, and at the mezzo level, for example, across the entire sport discipline.

Visual mapping in the form of a video, and less often photos, allows to gain insights into the specificity of one's movement and its aesthetic appearance alongside the overall body look and its surroundings. The specificity of one's own motion and personal appearance are the elements the exercising person wants to see on the screen. Similarly, other components of the activity effects (the results achieved, the parameters obtained) can also be subject to visualization. This happens due to the use of self-tracking applications, simulators, timers, heart rate monitors, etc. Data collected by these devices is analyzed and subsequently converted into a visualized form of maps, diagrams, tables, graphs, etc. The gathered information is subject to further analysis.

Visualization of training, and especially the visualization of motion in the form of a video, lies at the base of self-improvement. In some cases, it is enough to analyze the movement assisted by watching the film; in others, parameters and results analyses are included. Thus, qualitative analysis is sometimes supplemented by quantitative analysis. Improvement, which in most cases focuses on self-improvement, is based on the pursuit of perfection and accuracy interpreted individually and from one's own perspective.

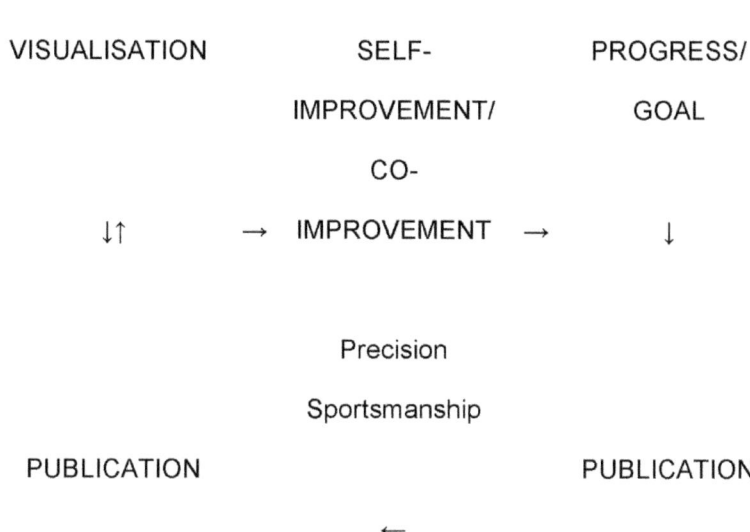

Figure 4.2.   Mediatization mechanisms of self-improvement and co-improvement.
Source: own elaboration.

It is the precision of mapping (e.g., someone else's instruction video or one's own movement), precision of refining details, and obtaining a comprehensive effect that is in line with the desired outcome, e.g., model effect. Visualization in the form of a moving image in HD quality allows one to refine the smallest details. In the absence of third-party (trainers, partners) support, and even when accompanied by others, achieving the ideal effect most often determines one's acceptance of the achieved result. This result may be relatively weak, but if it demonstrates progress for the exercising individual, it creates a sense of achievement. Fulfilling the conditions of the relative perfection of sportsmanship and aesthetic perfection, the created video material can be published to provide the exercising person with a source of social recognition and motivation. It may become the basis for creating a broader video material that will make progress far more visible in a longer time perspective. Such materials can potentially serve a source of knowledge, inspiration, motivation, and a point of reference for others. Thus, practicing sports aficionados can learn from one other and documented efforts can invite feedback. If the material included is seen as a novelty due to an innovative solution style, technique, method, or choreography, it has a great potential to become a forerunner of changes in a given technique, style, or even across the entire discipline. It can contribute to the transformation of a given form of physical activity and its popularity. It can also influence its new social meanings and inspire others to take up physical activity or choose it above other disciplines. In addition, it can bring the author material benefits directly (from advertising cooperation based on the published content) or indirectly (as a tool for the promotion of activities in the sports industry). In the latter case, the published material can turn the exercising person into an expert. In other words, independent training based on online materials and followed by publicizing the visual effects of one's development has the potential to make them not only an online expert, but a competent coach or adviser as well.

The described mediatization mechanism is revealed at a certain stage of sporting advancement, but it plays a significant role in initiating and educating beginners. Its drawback, both for beginners and advanced individuals, is the illusion that the level of precision, perfection, and sportsmanship achieved is objectively high. Due to the lack of participation of instructors, trainers, etc., in the training process, different ways of validating the achieved effects are necessary. They can comprise of shows, workshops, competitions, partner trainings, and consultations with other exercising individuals. However, not everyone takes advantage of them. To some respondents, acceptance received via social media is satisfactory and they usually resort to self-recording, self-analysis, and self-acceptance, seeing physical activity mainly as a source of pleasure, a way of spending free time, and taking care of themselves. They do not break records and do not attempt to exceed their limits, which would require cooperation with professionals. They, however, have the same ability to influence the shape and principles of their disciplines as well as the nature and popularity of their chosen physical activity. Above all, they take part in the process of peer, collective, and reciprocal learning. The process of their mutual education and improvement facilitates the development of disciplines, particularly those seen as relatively new. They emerge and are shaped in the present moment. It is a social process, facilitated by social media and aggregation media, and indirectly assisted by the technological possibilities allowing for a video creation, potentially by every exercising person.

MEDIATIZATION OF NICHE PHYSICAL ACTIVITIES

The presented research results on the mechanisms of mediatization significantly supplement the gap in the research on the broadly understood use of video cameras in physical activity and in research on the cultural and social dimensions of filming and publishing this type of video material online. The existing studies in this field are mainly related to ethnomethodology and psychology involving the use of video cameras, e.g., as part of the stimulated recall method.[25] As Susan Houge Mackenzie and John H. Kerr point out, due to the analysis of recordings of the respondents, they carried out studies in decision making in orienteering, social experience in mountain biking, the temporal dynamics of acrobatic activity, and psychological aspects of participation in whitewater adventure activities, among other studies.[26]

Previous research on physical activity with the use of video cameras—whether used spontaneously by sports enthusiasts or artificially introduced to physical activity of the investigated individuals to obtain research material—mainly concerns disciplines such as: mountaineering, surfing, cycling, mountain biking and hiking, hang gliding, skydiving, whitewater canoeing, street-racing, and extreme cycling.[27] Neither of these studies, however, attempted to explain the mediatizing mechanisms of the video camera use.

In the history of media development, the introduction of GoPro cameras in 2004 bore a great significance for mediatization and activities categories as "extreme sports have leant themselves to changed recording techniques for moving cameras with mobile subjects."[28] This triggered the emergence of similar, sometimes cheaper, micro-cameras modeled on GoPro (i.e., headcams), which have gained enormous popularity due to their light weight and dimensions, resistance (including waterproofing), and ease of attaching to the body and adjacent equipment. From the moment of their release, such video cameras were called sport cameras and they were first used by amateurs of action sports, extreme, and lifestyle sports. Due to the development of smartphones, video cameras began to gain the status of universal devices in some sport disciplines, and the live streaming fashion contributed to the publication of more and more amateur video content on the web. In light of the conducted research, video cameras are preferred mainly by fans of niche sports.

So far, research on the use of video cameras in physical activity has not been concerned with mediatizing mechanisms underlying their individual application and their socio-cultural consequences. The research results published hitherto confirm the implications of mediatization, but without penetrating deeper into the properties of media technology and mediated processes, which in the context of physical activity lead to multiple transformations. Closest to media research are studies on sports sub-cultures that recognize digital media as central for the development and popularity of sub-cultures, such as parkour[29] or surfing.[30] These studies, conducted within diverse paradigms and various sub-disciplines (from microsociology,[31] mobile video ethnography,[32] through psychology of physical activity and cultural studies, e.g., on the so-called video-velo-culture[33]), partially confirm the conclusions drawn from the media studies presented above, but indicate the existence of many gaps that research on mediatization has not yet addressed.

At the micro level, relevant studies reveal the importance of video cameras in documenting physical activity, and particularly their role in documenting users' progress.[34] We can see the motivational significance of the video camera presence itself, which, reaching back to the time when cameras were the dominating medium, was referred to as "Kodak courage."[35] However, the significance of a video recording for motion analysis purposes is negligible and if such application arises, it is mainly related to research practice rather than the activity undertaken on the amateurs' initiative. In terms of video recordings analysis, it is emphasized that, while video cameras allow individuals to visualize activity aspects previously unnoticed,[36] the importance of the footage taken by a third party cannot be overestimated.[37] The conclusions concerning the specifics of time management also emerge, i.e., spending time on media activity during physical activity is relatively long, if not longer than the time dedicated to the activity itself.[38] Sometimes video is used to communicate feelings and experiences,[39] an observation also confirmed by research on mediatization, and YouTube in particular serves as a platform for self-expression and identity-building within different sports sub-cultures.[40] In the light of the research on mediatization, YouTube proves to be primarily a platform for knowledge and sharing experience sometimes associated with running a business, as is the case among the researched paraprofessionals. Media saturation studies bring new arrangements pertaining to changes in the course and nature of physical activity at the individual level, and the consequences it has for the development of some sport disciplines.

At the mezzo level, researchers from related disciplines emphasize the importance of video production, often referred to as "participant-driven visual production,"[41]—for the development and popularization of sport disciplines. Studies published to date, however, lack detailed explanations of the development mechanisms. In terms of sports sub-cultures popularization, the importance of marketing is emphasized, although it is evident in the research of this volume, it does not apply to all researched respondents since amateurs' self-presentation may not be aimed at commercializing their sports activities.

The most relevant conclusions on the mediatization of physical activity were drawn by Paul Gilchrist and Belinda Wheaton based on the subject of "peer support and pedagogic interventions,"[42] which can be considered as an element of the mediatizing mechanism of self-improvement and co-improvement. Although they recognized the role of media technologies in (self) education, the need "to probe deeper (. . .) structures and constraints, that come into being technologies and the opportunities are distributed"[43] was expressed and the presented research addresses that need in the context of sport media saturation. The studies presented in this volume mainly include the findings on the use of video cameras embedded in smartphones, which replace or complement stand-alone cameras and condition the way the resulting video material is used, generating subsequent changes.

MEDIA SATURATION INVESTIGATION

Research on media saturation by digital cameras of niche forms of physical activity confirmed the dominant importance of smartphones, which are considered the technology of the first order. This, in turn, confirmed the conclusions derived from the research on the dominant forms of physical activity (running and gym workout). The video cameras built into smartphones are mainly used by amateurs and create constellations with other media technologies aided by hardware, software and mobile properties of smartphones. Cameras in smartphones and smartphones alone could be equipped with desired features, parameters (regarding functionality) to guarantee a certain quality of content. Paradoxically, and despite the existing conditions to increase their capabilities due to the available accessories, they are devoid of them. Therefore, technological saturation is based on the available functions of embedded digital cameras, which universally present in everyday life, show an increasingly paradoxical and sometimes changing nature. They become transparent and obvious, but become visible again to users whose sports practices are integrated with media practices.

Facilitated by the use of digital cameras, a processual saturation involving analysis, memorializing, communication, self-presentation, and promotion occurs. Qualitative analysis of processual saturation revealed the basic mechanisms of mediatization behind the use of video cameras: self-improvement and co-improvement, causing the transformation of certain forms of physical activity. The visual form of the content that is generated and often made available, entails aestheticization and deaestheticization, which concern both the form of the material being created and the elements of sports practice (e.g., the outfit or surroundings chosen for a photo or video, etc.). The consequence of the visual and social aspects of mediatization of amateur sport also leads to distinctive pressure that active individuals experience. It concerns, in some cases, the use of video recording technology during a workout, and in the case of paraprofessionals, the creation and use of video materials for promotional purposes. Once again, it has been demonstrated, that the excessive presence of media technologies in physical activity and the processes medi-

ated by it triggers resistance mechanisms. Therefore, partial media desaturation, evident among physically active individuals, requires closer exploration.

NOTES

1. In quantitative research, 6.1 percent of respondents declared their use while its position in the hierarchy of priority was ranked as seven out of nineteen of the indicated technologies.

2. Their application was declared in quantitative studies by 4.6 percent of respondents, but at the same time the GoPro-type camera was the fourth in the order (after the music player, smartphone, and Endomondo application), placing it as the most important to the physical activity being practiced; and ninth in the priority hierarchy out of nineteen technologies indicated.

3. Specifically, one runner and one gym goer pointed to GoPro-type cameras, while the smartphone camera was indicated by four individuals who engage in workouts.

4. Especially of young Poles, who constituted studied population, CBOS, *Aktywność Fizyczna Polaków* BS/129/2013. http://www.cbos.pl/SPISKOM.POL/2013/K_129_13.PDF (retrieved online).

5. For example, the assumption that, although theoretically certain disciplines can be practiced all year, weather conditions of the research location (Wrocław, Poland) are adequate only for a part of the year.

6. In conditions of moderate climate characteristic of Poland where research was conducted.

7. Paraprofessionals should be understood as amateurs, who partially and in some dimensions, professionalize their sporting activity, but they are not professional athletes.

8. The status is considered from the point of view of the research location (Poland).

9. Calisthenics is a relatively young discipline the representatives of which have founded a sports association in Poland and it is currently in the process of establishing its activity.

10. The research was carried out between September 2016–February 2017 and May–July 2017. It was not possible to conduct direct observation in all cases. At that time, the data obtained from the respondents or shared on the web were used. The visual materials provided by the respondents also varied in character and information appropriateness from the point of view of the research focus.

11. Observation was not carried out in the case of paragliding, classic horse riding, and western-style horse riding due to the lack of such possibility; and in the case of pole dancing, due to the lack of consent of the respondent. In those cases, video and photo materials delivered by respondents and/or additional material publicly available online were analyzed to supplement individual interviews.

12. Only in the case of paragliding a smartphone was not indicated as a device used for filming.

13. More about the changes in the course of training can be found in the following section.

14. More on the self-sufficiency thanks to media can be found further in this chapter.

15. The use of recording technology and the reception of the content created during exercise was declared by 5 respondents who were all paraprofessionals.

16. More on desaturation in chapter 5.

17. "(. . .) my trainer tells me it's good and when I record it I see that there are still some things I could improve," (female pole dancer).

18. Details related to the decision pertaining to selecting published materials are disclosed in further part of the study.

19. "It gives you an external kick (. . .); a group of fans pushes you to do better" (male fitness body builder); the comments have the character of advice and are motivational, i.e., "Listen, you made mistake like this here. Correct it next time" (male cross-fitter).

20. More on promotion and development of young disciplines due to video recording can be found later in this chapter.

21. Worse quality prevents noticing "minimal things, which sometimes is crucial" (female western-style horse riding).

22. E.g., in pole dance training only on one side of the body, "the better side," may lead to spine deformities.

23. This is declared by, i.e., the practitioners of disciplines such as calisthenics, fitness body building, mountain cycling, skiing, western-style horse riding, parkour, classic horse riding, ballroom dance.

24. In the case of parkour, video recording and publication transform the discipline on a deeper, different, often cultural level. In fact, video recording changes the philosophy on which this activity is based. In accordance with its rules, one practices parkour for themselves, to overcome adversity in life in general, and to stimulate self-improvement. Showing off one's achievements and challenges is seen as contradicting the key principles of this form of activity.

25. Susan Houge Mackenzie and John H. Kerr, "Head-mounted Cameras and Stimulated Recall in Qualitative Sport Research," *Qualitative Research in Sport, Exercise and Health* 4(1) (2012): 51–61.

26. Ibid., 60.

27. See the analysis of the state research in, e.g., Paul Gilchristand and Belinda Wheaton, "New Media Technologies in Lifestyle Sport," in *Digital Media Sport: Technology, Power and Culture in the Network Society*, ed. Brett Hutchins and David Rowe (New York: Routledge, 2013); Katrina Myrvang Brown, Rachel Dilley, and Keith Marshall, "Using a Head-mounted Video Camera to Understand Social Worlds and Experiences," *Sociological Research Online* 13(6), 1 (2008).

28. Eric Laurier, Barry Brown, and Moira McGregor, "Mediated Pedestrian Mobility: Walking and the Map App," *Mobilities* 11(1) (2016): 5.

29. E.g., Gilchrist and Wheaton, ibid.

30. E.g., Clifton Evers, "Researching Action Sport with a GoPro TM Camera: An Embodied and Emotional Mobile Video Tale of the Sea, Masculinity and Men-who-surf," in *Researching Embodied Sport: Exploring Movement Cultures*, ed. Ian Wellard (London: Routledge, 2015); Clifton Evers, "Masculinity, Sport and Mobile

Phones," in *The Routledge Companion to Mobile Media*, ed. Gerard Goggin and La-rissa Hjorth (London and New York: Routledge, 2014): 375–84.

31. Mike Lloyd,"On the Way to Cycle Rage: Disputed Mobile Formations," *Mo-bilities* 12(3) (2017): 4.

32. Justin Spinney, "A Chance to Catch a Breath: Using Mobile Video Ethnogra-phy in Cycling Research," *Mobilities* 6(2) (2011).

33. Eric Laurier, "Capturing Motion: Video Set-ups for Driving, Cycling and Walking," *The Handbook of Mobilities,* eds. Peter Adey, David Bissell, Kevin Hun-nam, Pete Merriman, Mimi Sheller (Abingdon: Taylor & Francis 2013): 6.

34. E.g., Gilchrist and Wheaton, ibid.

35. Kathleen Gasperini, "Kodak Courage." *Mountain Sport and Living*, January–February (1999), cited in Gilchrist and Wheaton, ibid., 43. In the analyses presented above, the phenomenon pertained to rowing and horse riding, but was of an inten-sive nature, and it did not play as significant role of "performing for the camera" as indicated by N. Dempsey.; Nicholas P. Dempsey, "Stimulated Recall Interview in eEthnography," *Qualitative Sociology* 33 (2010): 349–67.

36. Evers, Researching action sport. . ., 10.

37. Lloyd, ibid., 5.

38. Evers, ibid., 4.

39. Ibid.

40. Gilchrist and Wheaton, ibid.

41. Ibid., 4.

42. Ibid., 9.

43. Ibid., 12.

Chapter Five

Desaturation of Physical Activity

The results from the previous stages of the research indicate that one of the significant processes in physically active individuals is the partial and intentional abstention from using selected media technologies during exercise.[1] This discovery prompted further investigation about the reasons for participants' withdrawal from technology and about its implications for physical activity as a result of subsequent desaturation. Consequently, it seemed prudent to examine the specificities of particular activities that become devoid of media technology involvement.

To examine the phenomenon and in order to draw comparisons to the conclusions deriving from the earlier stages of the research, the subsequent analysis focused on participants engaging with the most popular sports disciplines, namely running and working out at the gym. Similarly, and with the focus on partial desaturation, participants who withdraw from using the most popular media technologies, i.e., music players and self-tracking applications, were selected for analysis.

The core method to investigate desaturation in comparison to findings offered in the previous chapters was dictated by the need to obtain first-person accounts of the sports aficionados. For that purpose, individual, in-depth, semi-structured interviews were adopted.[2] The respondents included individuals engaging in regular, purely amateur physical activity who withdraw from the use of media technologies at large during exercise. Each of the surveyed participants engaged in at least one of the aforementioned popular sports disciplines, i.e., running and/or working out at the gym, with the vast majority involved in more than one type of training (two–three on average).

The sample comprised of fifteen respondents of different ages (between 18–46 years old with the average of 32.8) and sexes (eight women and seven men). Wide age choice was dictated by the need to obtain highly varied data from individuals with diverse qualitative and quantitative experiences and circumstances. On the one hand, younger individuals (school and university age) have relatively less sports experience and financial resources to invest in media technologies, however, they show a greater interest in them.[3]

On the other hand, older individuals (above 26 years old),[4] grew up in different technological conditions, with less widespread access to the Internet, mobile devices, or digital technologies at large. While the survey shows they have less trust in technology,[5] they may have potentially greater sports experience and financial possibilities. Therefore, the inclusion of participants from two distinctive age groups facilitated the opportunity to obtain much more varied reflections and observations from the sample respondents.

TYPES OF MEDIA DESATURATION

The research revealed two main types of media desaturation: complete desaturation, seen as isolation; and relative, based on periodic (temporary) or span related (concerning selected technologies or processes mediated by them) withdrawal.

Complete Desaturation

Complete desaturation occurs when a physically active individual essentially does not use any media technologies during exercise and often refrains from engaging with technology prior or after the activity too. The only technologies present are possibly residual (these are few and not specifically dedicated to physical activity), and their use is sporadic. In other words, they are not used regularly or play a significant function for physical activity (i.e., a smartphone is within reach, but only in exceptional situations messages are viewed or a phone call is answered, with both instances unrelated to the training in progress). Physical activity is treated as an activity isolated from media technologies and mediated processes, but it is seen a complete isolation since multiple devices remain within the user's reach.

Within the research cohort, physical activity of six out of fifteen respondents was characterized by complete saturation. Among those six, one half did not use media technologies at all, while the other half of them abstained from using them over periods of time.

Complete desaturation can be defined by the desire to refrain from, eliminate technological excess, or avoid unnecessary interference during training, both in the material and processual sense. Individuals desaturating their physical activity most often indicate a physical interference of the equipment during exercise. The devices and accessories make the activity difficult and obstruct free movement. For example, wired headphones used during training may result in the forgoing of some exercises due to the potential danger of getting entangled in the audio cables or sub-optimal performance which in the long run can lead to health impairment (e.g., due to overstraining of particular vertebrae).

All in all, the respondents refrain from using many technologies purely out of convenience, for pragmatic reasons, to ensure freedom of movement and safety. In this context, the most notorious and undesired devices were smartphones, music players, and headphones with respondents perceiving them as totally unnecessary or posing difficulties for physical activity. This indicates media technologies are still insufficiently developed and unhandy while their accompanying accessories causing further hindrance (with headphones mentioned as the chief example).

Additionally, the costs of devices and accessories are still seen as high and the risk of damage, increased during the training sessions, also leads to abstention from using them. Singular usage attempts often leads to technical problems (i.e., with the GPS in self-tracking applications; insufficient capacity of the smartphone battery during long distances) as well as the need to carry the load of additional equipment to use the device (i.e., the requirement to engage with the GPS embedded in a smartphone to be able to use the key functions of a smartwatch).

In this context, technology is reflexively evaluated, and therefore, in no case, it becomes imperceptible or "transparent" to the user. The respondents' statements reveal a sense of externality and the unnatural nature of technology. Their desaturating reactions are driven by the desire to separate technology from their own body and their activities. Body and movement are a unity, in relation to which technology is external and additional, and often deemed unnecessary. In other words, its presence and use are treated as an undesirable interference. This also concerns the aspect of possible monitoring and external control. Only one respondent drew attention to the risk of either addiction to technology or the harmfulness of electromagnetic radiation, the absence of which becomes an incentive via desaturation:

"Honestly, it upset me a bit, because there was some lazy Saturday morning, for example, when I saw that I took 8 steps, that is to get two coffees and back to the bedroom, I can honestly say that I did not want someone to tell me how many steps I have to take every day or what to eat or not eat, so I just turned it off . . . and I rely on myself" (female, 40 years old).

In the processual dimension, a sense of waste of time resulting from the use of media technology was repeatedly mentioned. The respondents emphasized that technology always required sacrificing time before, during, or after train-ing, which further reinforced desaturation. Waste of time can refer to the tasks necessary for the preparation of the equipment prior to activity, including, for example, adequate battery charge or preparation of content, e.g., a playlist, downloading and entering data into the application, etc. The use of technol-ogy during the course of a workout also means that a significant amount of exercise time is devoted to interaction with the device (using the application, checking results, photos; interpersonal communication accompanying these activities, etc.). After the workout, time is dedicated to either data analysis or publication of content related to the activity, which can include searching for materials (e.g., music), and other tasks that, once again, seem unnecessary to the respondents. The potential waste of time can also result from unfulfilled expectations of greater automation of technologies (e.g., applications), par-ticularly in terms of having to remember about it (especially about starting it) and of many processes being carried out automatically:

"When I had to prepare myself for half an hour to run for half an hour, for ex-ample, 5 km, it made no sense to me at all. I just preferred to spend that half an hour running, rather than getting ready for it" (female, 40 years old).

Some of the respondents declare a sense of self-sufficiency during technology-free workouts, which most often arises from a great self-awareness of their bodies, their needs, and abilities, an observation unrelated to their age, but rather their attitude to physical activity. The goals of activity become of a less competitive character, i.e., its outcomes are not focused on numerical results, but on good health condition and overall well-being. The respondents declare, potentially resulting from discontinuing the use of the technologies, a greater awareness of their body, needs, and capabilities. They become more sensitive to the signals flowing from their bodies and more reflective and critical in relation to using technologies:

"It's nice to run just like that, when you feel, and based on how I feel, [decide], whether I can run harder or not. And based on what I feel, I can determine whether I'm running well or not running well. That's enough for me" (female, 33 years old).

It can be said then, that individuals desaturating their physical activity defi-nitely do not seek to professionalize it as they remain at a purely amateur level. As one of the respondents pointed out: "this is resting and the joy of doing it for myself. Nothing more than that" (female, 21 years old). Exercise becomes a means to an end itself and the time spent on it does not have to be filled with other activities, particularly if they demand mediation. Physical activity, therefore, becomes "pure" and undisturbed; it is private, personal and protected from unnecessary interferences:

"I consciously want to log out of those technologies as much as possible. It's a sort of detox, also technological" (male, 38 years old).

"When I go running I try to get rid of my phone; give my eyes, my brain a rest; and focus more on the motoric rather than on—let's say—what appears on the screen" (male, 28 years old).

Relative Desaturation

Based on the accounts of the majority of respondents (nine out of fifteen individuals), relative desaturation, either periodic, scope-based, or mixed, can be observed. Users abstain either from a particular or all media technologies for a period of time or choose to use only a limited number of media technologies. Sometimes both practices take place simultaneously. The reasons for the occurrence of relative desaturation vary.

In terms of periodic saturation, a given technology usually proves to be useful in certain circumstances (e.g., preparation for a competition), after which its significance decreases and is discontinued. In the investigated cohort, this most often applies to self-tracking applications such as Endomondo, purposefully used in new places and on new routes, but not in ordinary circumstances and familiar surroundings. Routine usage generates boredom and does not carry any substantial benefits, for example, in the form of important information, and therefore, users abandon technology. However, boredom with the exercises itself does not seem to concern them in particular. For individuals who give up technology, physical activity is engaging enough, so that they do need any special means of motivation to support their enthusiasm and energy, or to divert attention from the workout itself in order to persevere in the training. Simply speaking, they do not get bored while exercising and hence do not have to provide additional attractions.

In many cases, it is curiosity that determines the periodic application of technology. Testing[6] new technologies or their versions is interim and at random usually leads to conclusions that a given technology is unnecessary at a given time, circumstances, or in general.

Sometimes, and after a certain period of use, respondents conclude that they do not see the difference in training, regardless of the presence of technology. They also question the data or information obtained, e.g., measurements and estimates of self-tracking applications. Their attitude toward indications, calculations, or recommendations is rather skeptical and therefore they resort to simpler solutions (e.g., a simple watch to measure time instead of a smartphone with an application). The balance of gains and losses of the time investment, the burden on one's memory, and sometimes, the costs incurred prevails in favor of abandoning the technology.

Both in the material and processual dimensions, the respondents refute the myth of media omnipresence in every aspect of life. Most of them describe themselves as using media technology on a daily basis to a large or medium degree, but to a much smaller extent while exercising. Physical activity is differentiated from other daily activities by the lack of or a significant limitation of the presence and use of the technology. Exercises are seen as a kind of spatial and temporal enclave, allowing to concentrate on the movement itself. Smartphones are placed in changing room lockers, left at home, or silenced while other technologies are limited to a minimum or completely excluded.

MODELS OF USERS

The obtained results allow to distinguish three types of users who desaturate their physical activity: testers, sustainable practitioners, and liberated tech-slaves. A few respondents, however, seem to have featured two of those types combined.

Testers

Testers are a category characterized by relative desaturation. They use and dispose of particular media technologies after they personally investigated their functionality, application, and capabilities:

> "It was a matter of experiment: what could I do with a smartwatch?" (male, 34 years old).

They practically always abandon a tried-and-tested solution that either does not meet their expectations or begins to bore them in a short time span. While they take the opportunity to test new technologies, they also return to those already familiar ones to examine their new versions or features. They treat the use of technology as fun, a kind of additional attraction that can be given up at any moment. This mainly results from their perception of physical activity as the time devoted to themselves, their health, and pleasure. The use of technology stems from their curiosity and sometimes interest in technological novelties, e.g., a type of accessory or a new gadget. However, they do not have particular expectations of technology's impact on the course of their training, achieved results, etc. They treat it as a short-term form of increasing attractiveness of a workout, and an opportunity to discover another dimension of technological superfluity.

This applies mainly to self-tracking technologies, such as mobile applications for smartphones, heart rate monitors, or smartwatches as well as accompanying technologies, including music players and stationary technologies, e.g., training devices available in the gyms. Testers, assessing the examined technologies, question the sense of their long-term use and their credibility (e.g., credibility of provided data) while being aware of simpler and cheaper solutions (e.g., stopwatch instead of a smartphone with the application). They most often conclude that by using media technologies their physical activity neither gains anything, nor do they lose anything by giving it up. Testing, therefore, is a form of complementary entertainment, which is not accompanied by an in-depth reflection or conclusions related to the exercise.

Sustainable Practitioners

Sustainable practitioners are characterized by a particular attitude toward themselves and the surrounding environment during the exercises. First of all, they declare that they know themselves, their needs, and sporting abilities well. They trust their natural competences and therefore feel no need to support physical activity with technology. They show a large dose of skepticism toward its effectiveness, reliability, and the validity of use. Technology is definitely seen as an external, a bit foreign element to them:

"Let's say I'm in harmony with it, . . . with myself. I don't do anything for superficial reasons; to please someone or something" (female, 40 years old).

They do not use technology at all when they exercise (complete desaturation) or to a limited extent (relative desaturation). They want to engage in physical activity in harmony with themselves, but also feel connection to their environment, especially to nature. Being in harmony with oneself means listening to the needs of the body, maintaining moderation and balance that interference of intrusive technology can disturb. Activity is taken up only with their own well-being in mind and it is to constitute a kind of a rest and provide pleasure, which means that it must be characterized by freedom. To sustainable practitioners, the presence and use of technology limits this freedom and constitutes an unnecessary burden, of both a physical and mental nature:

"This creates a certain pressure that we create ourselves. And if you don't [have it], you just run and it's pure pleasure. You want to run faster, you run faster, you want to run more slowly, you run more slowly (. . .). And if I do not have a watch, I do not have Endomondo, then I do not focus on any external signals, how I am doing, I'm just enjoying running. I look around, admire nature . . ." (male, 46 years old).

In turn, maintaining a relationship with the environment during exercise means the lack of isolation of any of the senses, resulting in full awareness of the exercising person's surroundings and experiencing the pleasure from that particular connection. This particularly applies to nature, which is admired, provides rewarding experiences, makes movement more pleasant, and offers relaxation. Training itself is the main and sufficient source of joy and satisfaction, and the use of technology is perceived as risky. For some respondents, the risk consists of losing contact with oneself during exercise, which can hinder their ability to listen to their breathing and feel the pace of their heartbeat (when listening to music). It can also undermine their ability to assess their current condition and well-being (when following the indications of self-tracking applications). Some respondents were adamant that technology breaks one out of rhythm and hinders contact with their own bodies:

"When I hear someone wrote to me, I take a break. If I, let's say, let myself not take this break, then in my brain there is already that information that "oh! there is something waiting for me" and this often causes such a break from the rhythm I want to avoid, because I want to focus my mind on this one thing. Because when we are focused, we rest better. I need it and I care about it too" (female, 21 years old).

For some participants, the mere awareness of the presence of technology disturbs the rhythm of their exercise. In rare cases, they mention potential physical harm (radiation of devices, etc.) and the risk of addiction to technology. Ultimately, training is to offer "peace and quiet" to them, a moment of isolation from all issues and activities unrelated to their workout. Therefore, this specific cut-off is independent, conscious, and unmediated:

"I have a moment of such peace from all this, because at work I sit in front of the computer practically non-stop, and if I do not sit in front of it, I use the camera, almost all the time I have a smartphone, sometimes even two (. . .). If I spend time at home, the TV's usually on, and if not the TV, then music from YouTube is playing. If I go out somewhere, I often use the phone, so if I go to the gym, I have it just to check the time. And if I'm going to run, I leave it at home and I take a rest from it" (female, 23 years old).

The respondents notice possible losses resulting from abstention from technology, but most often they are negligible in comparison to the profits. Sometimes the thought about the possible use of technology during training leads to the fear of losing comfort achieved via desaturation, hence most of them do not see the need to test technologies or challenge the accepted practice:

"If I measured my distances, I would measure my time, I would have to improve my results all the time; and that would be . . . a big burden for me . . . above all psychological. I would have to compare, I would have to improve, and I do not want to do it!" (male, 38 years old).

Liberated Tech-slaves

"In running, there was a short period of time when I was fascinated by technology and I was trying to use everything I could, and now I'm actually leaving it" (female, 40 years old).

Liberated tech-slaves are individuals whose physical activity is characterized by complete or relative desaturation. For them, training assisted by media technologies used to be of great importance in the past, but it transformed their activity into something contrary to the idea that inspired the use of technology in the first place: to improve their condition, being in a good mood, and general well-being. Conscious desaturation in their case stemmed from the strive to avoid exercise-related stress. Therefore, they deliberately began to ignore the pressure to uphold their respective frequency, intensity, the course length, planned effects, etc. In terms of analytical applications and other monitoring devices (e.g., heart rate monitors), the users felt excessive control and lack of freedom. In most instances, physical activity ceased to give them pleasure and began to bear a sense of excessive discipline, regime or duty:

"There was a time when I thought it was fun, but then these were meticulous notes; heart rate, maximum, average and minimum heart rate . . . The time was also counted immediately. Well, in total, I started to create such training plans and to compare them . . . Once it came up to such extremes . . . that when [I was] gone for three days, I had to bring . . . a bike or even replace the bike with running. I had to have a heart rate monitor. And if I had three days without training [I had the thoughts] 'ah, my form will drop . . .' One could say that I was such a technology slave, of all these applications, and now I'm just totally indifferent" (male, 25 years old).

In the case of music players, the respondents pointed to excessive interference of the rhythm of the running or exercises, their instability and "chaotic nature" [sic]. There was also a limitation of the sense of security, resulting from being cut off from external factors, mainly noise, but in some cases also feelings brought by other senses:

"Putting on headphones made me feel like I lost orientation; as if I was stunned by something. I also had the need for my senses to be a 100 percent sharp" (female, 33 years old).

Individuals who fit into the model of liberated tech-slaves went through a similar path of sporting development based on the use of technology: from fun, achieved progress, and satisfaction, through the increasing internal and/or external pressure, up to the frustration resulting from dissatisfaction with themselves:

"I felt, at the time when I checked my results so often, that there was this pressure. And there were moments when I had a bad day and despite the fact that I wanted to run harder, I did not necessarily succeed, so some frustration was born. So, I think that, [now] that pressure is gone. And that's cool. People run because they want to run, for pleasure, not for results and for pressure, to be better and better" (female, 33 years old).

Subsequently, the exercising individuals realized the need to retreat from the existing conditions and this resulted either in a change in the sport discipline or in conscious media desaturation. This stage was characterized by activities aimed at restoring the initial satisfaction with exercise, and thus avoiding any forced motivation, competition with oneself or others, abandoning activities that were unsuitable for them and their abilities. Regardless of the particular motives, the change was possible chiefly due to the discontinuation of using media technologies:

"Getting rid of these Endomondo and all these time measurements brought some relaxation to the training regime. But also, at the moment, I feel I'm cutting myself more slack, that I do not have to do it that way . . .; that I will not complete the plan . . .? Maybe I won't . . . If I do not go for a run, I won't and so be it . . ." (male, 38 years old).

Due to the desaturation, liberated tech-slaves regained control over their training and, in a sense, themselves. They became more open to the environment—to what happens around them when they exercise and their surroundings. They regained freedom and thus, they decided to focus on following their own needs more and felt that working out gave them pleasure again (e.g., via choosing routes, places, or pace that perhaps did not guarantee the best results, but still gave them pleasure):

"I could run through hills, paddocks and heavier terrains . . . Normally, I would choose straight routes so that the time would be better so that I would not be stopped by the route, right? And when I run without [Endomondo], I just run . . . where my eyes tell me" (female, 40 years old).

Henceforth, the exercising individuals became rather cautious in the selection and application of technology, feeling its absence to a minimal degree, or rather, perceiving the return to using technology as a threat. Most of them have a very slight sense of any loss resulting from the desaturation of physical activity:

> "I do not want to give my consent, inside me, that I'm beginning to pay attention to the technique, that I want to speed up. If I want to be better, maybe I should think about some kind of competition . . . maybe take part in some tournament . . . And I do not want to do it!" (male, 38 years old).

As aforementioned, the described models most often reveal themselves in an unambiguous way, and less frequently the types are combined, where the combination usually comprised of a sustainable model with a tester or a liberated tech-slave. In the former case, testing practices usually reinforce the exercising individuals in following the sustainable model. In the latter, the change taking place in the course of technological liberation leads to the practice of a more sustainable approach.

In the research cohort, there was no case of the mixed model of the tester and the liberated tech-slave. This may derive from a potentially deeper change taking place in the exercising individuals underlined by the discontinuation of using technology. All of them were loyal and long-term users of technologies, and the abstention resulted in a strong sense unwillingness to make any further attempts at using media devices, even for testing purposes. The idea of a potential return to mediated solutions is often underlined by fear:

> ". . . it will again turn into such an unhealthy competition with myself. It will not be such a pleasure and it will not serve health but the other way round. . ." (male, 25 years old).

DESATURATION: GAINS AND LOSSES

As previously revealed, in terms of relative desaturation, the two most often eliminated technologies include self-tracking applications, mainly Endomondo (and other technologies with a similar purpose, e.g., heart rate monitors), and music players.

Self-trackers

In the case of Endomondo, the causes of desaturation are varied and correspond with the characteristics of three types of users. For testers, it is the depletion of the application's formula and its possibilities, or the lack of a direct translation of its use effects into training. For tech-slaves, a safety boundary is crossed and a sense of loss of control, pleasure, and freedom during training appears. Sustainable users, on the other hand, consider Endomondo and similar technologies as a means undermining their direct contact with themselves and/or the training environment.

Widely mentioned profits deriving from the abstention from Endomondo include regaining influence on the training regime, especially its intensity; better evaluation of one's abilities and subsequent priorities, growing awareness of inter-related factors within exercise, for example physical and mental abilities, including the influence of mood. Also, respondents pointed to gaining a sense of relaxation and turning training into a form of rest. In term of motivation, for some it lowered, which results in less intense training and weaker engagement, but it does not give rise to a sense of frustration. On the other hand, some respondents believe that excessive control demotivated them, so desaturation resulted not only in the return of pleasure, but also improved results determined by their own observations and simple measurements. By being able to listen to themselves, they plan their training better and achieve greater satisfaction. The advantages of tackling the new situation described above, are mirrored in accounts of individual users:

> "If I am totally focused on this rhythm of running, I think I am able to run a distance even faster than when . . . I think that I have a phone and I think that somewhere "there's that thing" that tells me, I ran that many kilometers, etc." (female, 33 years old).

The main disadvantages resulting from giving up Endomondo comprise of the loss of access to data and the inability to generate new data, allowing to draw conclusions. Subsequently, participants lose the possibility of improving their well-being with the achieved results. The archives and all collected documentation are also lost, so that they no longer have access to the history of their achievements alongside memories they sometimes miss. Another element they refer to is the loss of a "written proof" of their progress, the inability to follow the progress, and to even see it. Since the improvement of their fitness condition may take place quite slowly, it is difficult to notice it without the tools measuring and archiving data, which allow for subsequent analysis.

> "If I did something regularly and if I have this recorded, it makes me happy, just looking at the saved table . . . that I was running three times a week here and I was consistent and I have it, so to speak, in writing . . ." (female, 40 years old).

Music Players

Desaturation in the context of music players was dictated by similar reasons to those given for the abstention from self-trackers: music posed no meaning and listening to it created a sense of disruption for the course of training. Therefore, inversed mechanisms governing media saturation processes of listening technology of runners and gym goers can be observed. While they sought to cut off from the environment and escape from their own problems via mental-physical multitasking and thus generating a type of a tension, desaturating individuals abandon these technologies to gain or regain contact with their surroundings and themselves, achieving a mental and physical unity and a subsequent feeling of relaxation.

The main advantages of desaturation in this context refer to having a better command of one's own body through observation and listening to one's breathing and heartbeat. Thus, training becomes more harmonious in character. It is not artificially modified and therefore it poses no discomfort to the exercising individuals. "Listening to the real world" is another key argument mentioned, as it gives the respondents a greater sense of security and peace. Through observation, they become more aware of their surroundings and take pleasure from that; therefore, they consciously choose to resign from "cutting off" or even being "stunned." The biggest disadvantage, however, is the loss of motivation, arising especially in crisis situations, such as the end of a training session and the moment of exhaustion and the subsequent weariness. These shortcomings, however, appear to be insufficient for the respondents to permanently return to the use of music players.

Regardless of the type of media technology, and in the context of both the quantitative and qualitative dimension of the perceived losses, the respondents usually do not change the discipline or form of activity in which they participate.[7] They remain consistent in their decisions regarding desaturation, whether it is the complete or the relative type. They become more aware, considerate, or even critical, and they pursue their activity according to their own needs. To them, physical activity is completely or almost unmediated and this applies to the non-publishing of training materials, too. Exercises fulfill their function when they are not mediated or hybrid, and when they are a means to an end themselves; when "running is the most important" and it is not about "showing yourself off through running" (male, 44 years old), or other goals.

CURRENT SITUATION AND PERSPECTIVES

In the context of the process governing media desaturation of physical activity in its diverse form and intensity, it is important to assess whether media desaturation entails its demediatization. In general, amateurs' physical activity does not result in demediatization since they still use media technologies. In other words, their activity is saturated by media technologies, and thus it is mediatized. However, in the context of individual desaturation models, different variants of relationships with the media technologies can be observed and therefore, similarly to some aspects of mediatization, possible demediatization on the individual level may occur. It mainly involves the transformation of a given activity due to the abstention from the use of media technologies. Regarding testers, a rather shallow relationship with the media can be observed, resulting in the lack of deeper transformation of physical activity. Therefore, it is difficult to debate mediatization in this case, and consequently, demediatization as a result of desaturation. On the other hand, abstention from media technologies (permanent or changeable) of sustainable users does not lead to direct transformations of physical activity under the influence of the media and a reverse process can be observed. It is the lack of media usage (complete or relative desaturation) combined with the high awareness of their function, importance, and effects, that causes physical activity to proceed in that particular direction, and not otherwise. Conscious isolation from media technologies affects physical activity and it changes based on contact with oneself and the environment, which becomes undisturbed and unmediated. Desaturation, therefore, indirectly transforms the physical activity of sustainable users, who consciously abstain from using media technologies.

The deepest desaturation and, de facto, demediatization changes are observed in the liberated tech-slaves. Their intense use of media technologies led to strong mediatization on the individual level and thus to changes in the form and nature of physical activity.[8] In the course of events and unsatisfactory transformations, desaturation took place, but so did demediatization, since the resignation from the media triggered the aforementioned change. However, it did not result in a return to the original state, preceding the stage of strong mediatization. A new variant of behavior has developed: an isolation model (sometimes close to sustainable) based on negative experiences and hence more reflective and restrictive. Physical activity ceased to be saturated and mediatized, and became additionally subjected to new rules of conduct. Henceforth, the training individuals not only avoid technology, but are also more conscious of it. Since reflexivity and criticism characterize liberated tech-slaves, they are aware of its advantages and disadvantages and are more cautious about any additions to training, including novelties.

From the perspective of the activity itself, demediatization leads to its change into amateur and recreational; runners and gym goers return to their original methods, principles, and attitudes, which makes these activities acquire a pure, undisturbed and definitely one-dimensional character through desaturation practices. All training is to serve the individual; it is supposed to result in well-being and thus does not lead to the challenge of one's limits.

At present, the obtained results on media desaturation of physical activity can hardly be referred to other studies since there have been no comparative study carried out to date. Until now, the process of demediatization has only been alluded to and remains at the level of theoretical reflections.

Research on the media desaturation of physical activity will undoubtedly require continuation and extension of its scope, including the inclusion of the population of physically passive individuals (permanently or temporarily) and examining the relationship between the lack of physical activity and the use or non-use (so-called non-users study) of media technologies in this area of everyday life.

The next emerging area is unquestionably the issue of media desaturation of various other dimensions of everyday life, which are not isolated from physical activity. Therefore, there is a necessity of an integrated approach to the study of media saturation and desaturation of everyday life as such, taking into account the entire array of media technologies and the configurations they create.

NOTES

1. However, the search for candidates to conduct interviews and observations in previous stages of the research revealed the existence of a population of individuals who completely abandon using media technologies during physical activity, either commencing when they take up the activity or after a certain period of time.

2. The interviews were carried out between June and July 2017.

3. The current data referred to in chapter 2 and appendix 1 indicate that fact.

4. Individuals not yet researched under the research project presented in this volume.

5. Appendix 1.

6. The characterization of the tester user model may be found in further parts of the chapter.

7. It has to be taken into consideration that, as part of the presented research, only individuals physically active were surveyed. That does not include individuals who used to be active and are currently passive; who might have resigned from physical activity due to the effects of the media saturation of their physical activity and they would require a separate analysis.

8. The results obtained earlier and presented in chapter 4, also indicated mediatization on the socio-cultural level, e.g., the change of a character of particular sport disciplines.

Conclusion

Technologies and Physical Activity Mediatizing Processes

This volume identifies the mechanisms governing mediatization through transformations on the micro and mezzo level and at the cross-section of individual and collective processes. To achieve that, three spheres of physical activity and their interrelations have been analyzed: personal, social, and technological. The quantitative examination of media saturation aspects allowed for assessing the significance of media technologies' presence and usage on mediatization. The subsequent analysis of the quality of saturation demonstrated conditioning of mediatization occurrence by media properties and generated mechanisms.

Research on media saturation of physical activity revealed that, despite the wide range of available and generally used technologies, the degree of technological saturation is low in comparison to the processual saturation, which is moderately high. This means that during physical activity, individuals perform relatively many different tasks and actions with the use of a small number of technologies. The availability of a wide spectrum of technologies, however, is not without significance. They serve as a vast source of means and possibilities from which users can choose and adapt to their sport disciplines and personal needs determined by their level of fitness development. Certain technologies interweave with selected forms of movement, resulting in their transformation. Although the scope of media content used is wide: from texts, photos, films, numerical statistics, to music, audiobooks, less often radio or television programs, it is not the properties of specific content format that chiefly determine the possibilities of the mutual media-physical activity conversion. The change is mainly based on the properties of technology. Convergence results in the content acquisition of a multimedia character. It flows between different platforms and is in a state of constant forming. On its own, however, it does not play as significant a role.

It is the properties of the tools used to generate, alter, archive, and dissemi-nate content combined with particular processes of technology application in practice that generate mediatization. This is evident in the sensual nature of the listening technologies, including the sensation of technology-facilitated touch (e.g., headphones in one's ears) which is enough to transform the sport activity. The mediated multi-sensory experience causes the training to undergo significant metamorphosis.

In addition, while the physical activity-oriented media content continu-ously evolves, it is chiefly the technology that has recently undergone radical changes. During the pre-mobile and pre-Internet era, content on physical activity was very restricted to, e.g., keeping training diaries instead of track-ers; or to single photos taken mainly by others instead of selfies and videos made with one's own smartphone. Circulation of these materials was very limited, if it took place at all. Its significance for the community practicing certain forms of physical activity was equally negligible. The widespread use of portable media devices based on the digital infrastructure has changed the practices of amateur sports individuals and this sphere of contemporary life. It provided opportunities to create and share content that is both individual, private, intimate, and shared, social, and thus, transformable.

Parameterization of studies on mediatization forces the research to go be-yond content analysis. The research to date has strongly focused on how me-diatization is socially produced: how the flow of media content results in the construction of the socially shared world. Meanwhile, it is necessary to un-derstand how mediation is performed through consumption, in other words, to understand the processes governing the use of media technologies at an individual and diversified collective levels. The media production (mainly production of content) and the consumption (not only of content, but mainly of media tools and infrastructures) condition contemporary mediatization. It occurs due to the material properties of the media and the digital constella-tions that encompass relationships between different media platforms. It is also shaped by the relationships developed between users, technologies, and content. In the context of physical activity, the qualitative change is driven by the particular spectrum of technology and the degree of technological satura-tion, resulting with the subsequent implementation of mediated processes.

In sports, technologies were already present with stopwatches and counters among the most popular. Simulators and all types of calculators initiated the implementation of various types of machines in sport, which henceforth not only made measurements and allowed to carry out analyses (mainly based on users' own calculations), track progress, and plan subse-quent trainings, but they began to have a much more intense impact on the individual units of activity, e.g., a series of exercises, imposing a specific tempo, or providing motivating data. However, only with the advent of digital technologies and the growing availability of mobile media, sports technologies have become versatile, widespread, and over time, highly intrusive. Increasingly, their functioning relied on operating large resources: raw data, but also processed information. The escalation of media technologies' usage in physical activity stems not only from accessibility and strong needs of the exercise enthusiasts, but also of an emerging fashion. For example, jogging while listening to the music through headphones. At first, it was enabled by a Walkman, and later via new generations of music players. The fashion for self-trackers and sharing results in social media prompting similar mechanisms via mobile applications. Also, the widespread availability of technology resulting from affordable prices, ergonomics, and integration of many functionalities in hand-held devices fostered widening the spectrum of processes. Technologies specially dedicated to active individuals, including sports cameras, have started to appear while universal, converged multi-functional devices such as smartphones, have gained "sports" functionality. They found application in physical activity, as in any other area of everyday life that undergoes mediatization. As a result, concretization of common patterns of contemporary, mediatized culture, e.g., partial self-isolation; quantification of activity, documenting, and visualization of communication can be observed in amateur sport.

In that context, universal and multi-functional technologies dominate among young individuals and they can be used in many different activities. The technologies that are "always with us," accompanying most aspects of our everyday life, include smartphones and music players. They have a very large number of purposes, but mostly they are related to mobility and can accompany individuals moving across space, not only in sport. Music players accompany listeners engaged in daily activity (moving from one point to another, e.g., in a city), which serves the purpose of filling their time, enriching it, giving it new dimensions (physically: leading to moderating movement, and mentally: by facilitating thoughts through i.e., social isolation). The smartphone allows users to stay in touch, create and receive messages regardless of distance, stationary means of communication (computer, landline telephone etc.), and the user's location changes. Above all, it multiplies non-interpersonal functions, including analytical or archiving capacities.

Research on media saturation, however, shows that despite the universalization of technology, mediatization is not a homogeneous phenomenon. Its specificity cannot be generalized to the whole area of amateur sport or physical activity since it's expressed in a diversified manner. This confirms Friedrich Krotz's thesis that "it is not the differentiation of media that changes conditions of communication, it is the fact that individuals use the different existing technologies as media and thus communicate differently and con-struct different realities."[1] In line with that, Sonia Livingstone and Peter Lunt claimed that mediatization adopts a different course across different areas; in addition, within one particular area different ways and dimensions of media-tization can be observed. [2]

According to the conducted research, mediatization results in specific me-dia and sports worlds emergence. These worlds can involve both individuals engaging in particular forms of activity as well as those who use the particu-lar technologies. These worlds are intertwined, but the dominant, universal sports and media world differs from niche worlds. Technologies commonly used (smartphones, music players) mediatize mainly on the individual level and hence, they are responsible for micro-mediatization of sport, transform-ing it into hybrid activity, related to the grammar of new technologies: partly dependent on it, but also affecting its changes. Technologies used by a small percentage of physically active individuals mediatize deeper, both at the individual and social level, determining the transformation of activities and changing the forms of movement or entire sport disciplines. Popular technolo-gies and popular disciplines, similarly to niche technologies and niche sports, adhere to each other, and these relationships generate further dependencies and transformations. In the context of physical activity, niche technologies such as personal cameras are used at a higher level of sporting advancement, represent higher demands, which users set for themselves, but also for others, resulting in sport disciplines' dynamic development. Popular disciplines (run-ning, gym exercises) are less demanding (in terms of finances, organization, and competencies) and less complex in their principles, way of practicing, which makes them less flexible and thus less susceptible to mezzo-changes. They are also characterized by lower technological sophistication of individu-als who engage in those sports. However, it does not change the fact that their transformational impact is very strong at the micro level. Niche disciplines are often specific (in financial, inventory, organizational sense) and their ac-cessibility and popularity are lower in comparison to popular sports. They are, however, characterized by greater high-tech flexibility and openness to niche technologies, which lead to their popularization and social, cultural, and economic change.

However, it must not be forgotten that in the era of convergence, technolo-gies, and processes intertwine. In the media environment, structures and prac-tices are networked. Flexible, integrative, and multifunctional technologies lead the way to change on a mass scale. Media technologies used in physical activity serve all senses and operate on various levels: a music player pro-vides sound, a camera allows visualization using static and moving pictures, and a tracker operates on numerical data, providing both text, visual, and audio materials. Also, the generated content is subject to multimedia circulation through the use of social media platforms, which chiefly serve as a one-to-one and one-to-many communication tool. Smartphonization contributes to that to the highest degree. Smartphonization refers to all aspects of everyday life:

> "This is our life now: strongly shaped by the detailed design of the smartphone handset; by its precise manifest of sensors, actuators, processors and antennae; by the protocols that govern its connection to the various networks around us by the user interface conventions that guide our interaction with its applications and services; and by the strategies and business models adopted by the enterprises that produce them."[3]

Due to its handiness, versatility, and multi-functionality, the smartphone appears as a meta-medium into which diverse hardware and software are integrated. In such a complex and consolidated environment, the mediatization of physical activity occurs.

The conducted research reveals a highly paradoxical nature of media technologies. Due to their presence, some aspects of human activity become visible, more concrete, become detectable, while technologies seem to "disappear" from users' sight. Media technologies develop into obvious objects with users so accustomed their presence that they become "transparent," and almost "invisible." This results from their strong integration with everyday activities, habits, as well as practices. They penetrate everyday routines, structure them, enable self-management, and self-optimization at times. Technologies become ordinary, just as the activities undertaken are common, nondistinctive, and "integrated into everyday life as part of ordinary, daily routines."[4]

The users are more aware of the implemented, mediated processes than of the presence and application of the technologies used. Only oversaturation results in them becoming conscious of the technological excess. Saturation has a purely material appearance, manifesting itself in a sense of physical weight, but also as the effects of the excess of mediated processes. The users isolate themselves from processes that affect the nature of their physical activity. However, before it happens, they consent to a strong saturation of their everyday life with media technologies. Thus, the importance of media technologies in physical activity completes a circle: from their absence or very low significance, through the convergence of sports and media activities, to the return to pure, unmediated, nontechnologized physical activity. Consequently, the changes in the perception of technology by users follow a circle, too: from visibility, resulting from novelty, new possibilities, and evolving needs, through invisibility, resulting from strong saturation, to visibility again, arising from oversaturation and its consequences, which is accompanied by deepened reflexivity.

The research has revealed that the spectrum of media technologies used in physical activity is very wide, but most technologies are niche in character. Therefore, it is necessary to investigate whether it resulted from the technologies not meeting the users' expectations; their poor adaptation capabilities to the needs of exercising individuals, or perhaps they limited ability to fit many forms of activity. For the respondents, the simplicity of technology is significant, not its sophistication, and they tend to favor minimalism over the richness of design and functionalities. This does not mean that numerous functionalities are not used in other circumstances, but physical activity does not inspire that. Hence, it has been revealed that there were no individuals who could be perceived as flagship examples of the Quantified Self movement members.[5] While some of them declared episodes or periods strongly focused on subordinating their lives to quantifying technologies, it was the pursuit of practicing sports in a pure and undisturbed form that freed them from the use of such technologies. Physical activity is seen as a simple activity in its foundations and implementation, and therefore, the accompanying technologies should also be "simple." They have to fulfill basic functions, not burden the user (physically and mentally), and bear minimum requirements for their usage. Respondents' criticism indicate that the imperfection of technology and maladjustment to expectations still exist. The devices (especially with accessories) are perpetually seen as too heavy, bulky, or even dangerous (e.g., tangled headphone cables may cause physical injuries), susceptible to damage, with limited use possibilities (memory space and time—mainly due to insufficient battery life). Despite the convergence of the content, the specificity of the devices leads to their divergence, which is seen as impractical, and even tiring. All in all, physical activity is one of many areas of dissemination of media technologies alongside their specialization and convergence of mediated processes.

As aforementioned, universalization of technology applications makes it obvious and "transparent." For example, smartphone, as a multifunctional device, has the ability to integrate subsequent areas of activity and spheres of human life. Hence, smartphonization of life appears to be the main topic of mediatization.

> "The ubiquitous smartphone can be understood as both an indicator of mediatization and as a communications device whose distinctive pattern of affordances and often highly personal practices of usage contribute to its intensification. (. . .) The smartphone as an object of material culture is surely a significant aspect of mediatization. In its design, development, and use, it is a powerful accelerator of that process, while its rapidly globalizing adoption is an undeniable indicator of the expanding presence of mediatization."[6]

In the context of sports activity, technology constantly evolves to address new users' expectations. Various solutions are offered to integrate functions to a higher degree and processes, e.g., applications for individuals practicing sports go hand-in-hand with applications related to diet, medical treatment, and broadly understood well-being. Thus, technology universalization is reinforced and the scale of mediatization is extended, but its depth increases to a lesser extent. On the other hand, non-universal technologies offer greater specialization and paraprofessional possibilities. By reaching narrower groups, they mediatize them more intensely and to a deeper extent.

MICRO-MECHANISMS AND MEZZO-MECHANISMS OF MEDIATIZATION OF PHYSICAL ACTIVITY

The research revealed the main micro- and mezzo-mechanisms of mediatization resulting from the qualitative and quantitative saturation of the media. Thus, changes in the media saturation can be perceived as conducive to mediatization since they reinforce it, sometimes condition it, both in terms of materiality of technology and processuality of action.

Media technology use transforms physical and mental activity at the individual level and changes amateur sport in many dimensions at the social level. It is at the micro level that both the main reasons for doing sports and the rationale for the use of media technologies appear. For young individuals, personal needs dominate, mainly related to physical elements (attention to fitness, well-being, appearance, better overall health condition), although they do not appear in a complete isolation from other requirements (such as satisfying the need for self-reflection and emotional self-regulation). Media technologies are introduced into training sessions for similar purposes. At the same time, they bring additional elements to training by, for example, contributing to mental and social isolation. The users cut themselves off from their body (e.g., the sounds of loud breathing) and mind to immerse intensely in training. They do not want to think about certain things, and above all, they want to avoid any potential disruption from the external environment. Workout is the time to cut off from other daily activities, from other places, and other individuals. It is a kind of activity enclave. Media technologies allow them to generate a sanctuary in two dimensions: physical and symbolic. It has been shown, however, that contradictions and paradoxes accompany this process. On the one hand, users favor multitasking and efficiency; on the other, they desire to return to themselves and to treat activities as natural, i.e., to engage in movement for the sake of it with. Regardless of their intentions, media technologies are at the core of those mutually exclusive attitudes.

In addition, the study revealed a series of micro- and mezzo-mechanisms, which are based on the growing importance of media technologies use. Micro-mechanisms, in addition to that isolation, include e.g., mobilizing oneself and increasing the efficiency of workouts, modifying workouts in the short- and long-term, as well as general self-improvement. The macro-mechanisms include co-development of forms of activity, aestheticization of physical activity and social communication, self-presentation (of non-commercial nature), and promotion (for commercial purposes). The results show a strong individualization in the utilization of technology. From a wide spectrum of available options, users create their own constellations of platforms that are interrelated to various degrees. They receive and create media content individually, which coincides with individual training (often devoid of partners, and above all, trainers or instructors, as well as limited to the anonymous company of random individuals). The mediatized physical activity is strongly personalized and individualized, at times to such an extent that the development is based on self-education with the use of the new media. This leads to the assessment of the degree of one's own progress based on social media-facilitated self-criticism and self-evaluation, which poses multidimensional risks. On the one hand, insufficient self-awareness, resulting from reciprocal learning on the web, entails the risk of duplicating mistakes, but also broadening the collective unconsciousness about the alleged progress and correctness. It is associated with an increased risk of health deterioration, and, in extreme sports, even one's life. As the importance of prosumption and commercialization of activity via social media increases, the problem becomes even more severe. Individuals educating and promoting themselves, a discipline or physical activity at large, derive profits from being recognized as experts and authority figures, which is not always the case. Thus, amateur sports reveal mechanisms that we can observe in other spheres of social life, such as politics, culture, or business. These include a decrease in the importance of direct contact with a specialist in a given field and the preference for pro-ams,[7] as well as the general decline in search for unmediated contact with another person in public space.

The mediatization of amateur sport began to gain momentum not so much due to the use of ever-diverging devices, but due to the mediation of uncountable processes and the ever-stronger convergence of everyday activities at large. From the initial desire to enrich and expand one's own capabilities during movement alongside the growing number of technology users, the collective social implications of devices and applications use in various forms of physical activity have become apparent. The potential of many technologies, combined with social media and exploited in the context of disciplines, have resulted in new sports identities, specificity, rules, and dimensions. For example, personal video cameras resulted in the emergence and development of new forms of physical activity that previously were often not featured in traditional media; hence, if it were not for the new media, those new activities would probably not become widely known. All in all, amateur practices related to well-established sports disciplines have undergone and are still undergoing transformations and gaining new dimensions: social, educational, and commercial; thus, amateur sport is constantly becoming anew.

The visual nature of social media enforces the aestheticization of the created content, and, subsequently, the presented physical activity. It is worth noting that physical activity in itself is a very attractive subject of content, and therefore exposed to ever-growing intensity of prosumption and commercialization. Visualization is an important, bilateral mechanism, observed both at the micro and mezzo level. Visualizing the results of the workout, the captured image of oneself, the image of the activity and its environment, play a crucial role in the individual fitness development as well as in socialization of sport, which contribute to the arrival of other solutions serving the discussed visualization. The bilateral aspect applies also to the audial dimension on the individual level: while music influences the course of a workout, the exercise dictates the selection of tunes. Additionally, using audio devices in sport influences changes in technologies and media content (in the designed equipment, applications, the created repertoire, dedicated to physical activity).

Movement, relocating, particularly across large urban space, often predestines the use of technologies for cocooning,[8] enabling isolation, which can be seen as a sign of disregard for others. Both cocooning and phubbing[9] have been observed in amateur sport, but these are not the main mechanisms that mediatize physical activity. The primary reason behind the application of media technologies in physical activity stems from the strive for efficiency, improvement of achievements, and results in the form of changes in appearance or well-being. Physical activity is expected to bring a particular effect and to achieve it, the users listen to motivating music, use trackers, cameras, and video cameras, and often other media technologies that integrate with social media. A strong focus on efficiency sometimes leads to the distorted pursuit of one's own well-being, resulting in frustration, dissatisfaction, and, at times, a deterioration of motivation and results, which leads not only to a decrease in effectiveness but also to the abandonment of its pursuit. This reversal of order results in a profound shift in focus, from effectiveness to the pursuit of pleasure and freedom.

Mediatized physical activity is characterized by strong convergence. On the one hand, a workout strongly integrates physical and mental elements within its boundaries, on the other, both of these integrated spheres are connected and transformed by media technology. Deliberate planning, analyzing, and reflecting on everyday life, which take place during the workout, are strongly connected to and influenced by accompanying music. Also, creating media content, publishing, discussing, and sharing it, often before, during, and after training, make that sports activity socially-oriented, and in the case of paraprofessionals prosumed: co-produced and co-consumed. Thus, mediatized amateur sport converges various spheres of life: work and leisure, education and entertainment, responsibilities and free time. The convergence of these elements can lead to the users feeling overloaded, which results in desaturation, the aim of which is to restore the blurred borders again. It seems there is a strong desire to "purify" physical activity from disruptive elements, which mainly include technologically mediated processes. Users decide to completely isolate, temporarily resign, or partially "cut out" the media technology: they give up selected processes or technologies, or their particular functions. It is also worth noting that desaturation can be initiated at the mezzo level, e.g., in surfing, where the use of cameras and mobile technologies that locate users is perceived as a threat to the identity of the discipline, due to the risk of revealing the location of the trainings (surf spot secrecy). [10]

In the context of mediated processes, contradictions emerge at times. They may concern the nature of media technologies or pertain to the implications that their use brings. For example, the processes of listening to music seem to be of particularly ambivalent, isolating-integrating nature: while isolating socially (from other individuals) and personally (from oneself, one's own physical symptoms), they facilitate the internal integration of body and mind. Similarly, the quantitative-demotivating trackers demonstrate contradictions: on the one hand, they quantify the activity, serving the purpose of improving efficiency and satisfaction; on the other—they can take away the pleasure from doing sports, discourage further pursuits, and eventually lead to passiveness. The technologies often generate a kind of internal division, manifested in contradicting statements of the respondents.

Paradoxes can also be observed in the social dimension: while disciplines and forms of movement develop, popularize, and even commercialize through the use of media technologies, this development poses a threat of "spoiling" them, compromising their uniqueness, and even the basis of one's identity—such is the case with parkour. The promotion of inadequate attitudes, practices, and behaviors brings a risk of degeneration of that discipline and amateur sport as such. The essence of physical activity lies in the effort aiming to improve or maintain a person's general well-being: it is chiefly supposed to serve that individual, with the potential element of competition. Meanwhile, social co-shaping of forms of movement, focused on promotion or commercialization by amateurs of physical activity, are not present in its original, nonmediatized version. Once mediatized, an activity becomes a hybrid subjected to those elements' interaction with one another, while each participant can possibility play a role in this transformation. As a result, modulated, reshaped, and transformed physical activity is no longer based only on a movement aimed at benefitting the body and possibly the mind, too. It becomes a converged action of both body and technology alongside its operational processes, and thus its contribution expands into a wide scope of individual and social goals.

The mind is perceived as responsible for communication with oneself, with the device, and with others, while the body works: it performs the physical activity as well as contributes to interactive communication: with the device, the content (data, information), and other individuals. Interactive communication is the main mediator of the undergoing change. Media technology co-participates in the user's activity, but very often it neither involves in interpersonal communication nor in communication with standardized content, or its engagement is minimal. Most processes do not have a communicative character in their traditional sense as it is of either an interactive or a passive nature. This type of communication mediates the largest number of processes carried out in the course of physical activity. It also plays a key role in modifying the activity at the micro level. Saturation with the processes of interactive communication, which to some extent is also passive, generates a number of mediatization mechanisms. These mechanisms constitute models of mediatization, both in the processual dimension (which explains the study of usage models), and in the structural dimension (which is explained by the study of the technologies and their properties). Their consequences result in changes that can be observed in the world of broadly defined sport. One of them is the democratization of sport, activity ("everyone" can be active, "everyone" can be a coach, in sport, everyone is equal) reinforced by "peer support and pedagogic interventions."[11] Such beliefs arise from the access to educational materials as well as the possibility to create and publish them freely. Self-education, disintermediation of instruction and coaching processes, optionally peer co-education, are accompanied by self-expression and building one's own image. Thus, physical activity appears as a field of entrepreneurialism. "Physical capital, then, becomes cultural and economic capital."[12] In turn, along with the development of disciplines, especially the emerging and niche ones, change of their rules and identity building, particular cultures or sub-cultures are formed. Their development, growth of popularity, and potential commercialization are determined by communication with the new technologies.

When considering the results of the study in the light of previous studies on the mediatization of sport, it should be stressed first of all that this area has been dominated by studies on the mediatization of professional sport, and in addition, they mainly concern traditional media, especially television. They are primarily part of the institutional approach. These include the works of Kirsten Frandsen, [13] Thomas Birkner and Daniel Nölleke, [14] Andrew Billings, [15] and David Rowe. [16] The development of digital media has led to an increased interest of researchers of professional sports (e.g., Yair Galily, [17] Gerard Goggin [18]), also looking at sport from a cultural perspective (e.g., Jimmy Sanderson [19]), but above from an economic perspective (e.g., Brett Hutchins and David Rowe [20]).

The area of mediatization of amateur sport or, more broadly, physical activity, and even more so mediatization by means of digital media technologies, is only just beginning to be analyzed. So far, few studies have been published in this area. The world of professional sport, synergistically integrated with traditional media, and the world of amateur sport, in which new media dominate, despite strong links and inspirations, are subject to mediatization to a different degree and on the basis of different mechanisms, which are difficult to compare with each other. The issue of the importance of media in amateur sport can be found in the studies mentioned in the volume, which have been published so far on the basis of ethnography and cultural anthropology, psychology, physiology, or a broadly understood methodology of humanities and social research. These studies focus on narrow areas, such as the use of cameras in surfing, or consider widely the importance of selected technologies in everyday life (e.g., listening technologies in motion). The reader can read about the complementarity or possible discrepancies in the results of each study in the concluding parts of chapters three, four, and five. The contribution of this volume should be seen in explaining the purely media aspects of the phenomena: the significance of the features of technology, their relations with users, the course of processes, and the way multi-level mechanisms of mediatization are developed. Volume combines the problems that so far have been spread between many paradigms and disciplines thanks to the proposed methodology of research on media saturation, at the same time inscribing it into the theory of mediatization. The research carried out undoubtedly develops a technological approach in research on mediatization.

The article by S. Lombork and K. Frandsen, which has been mentioned several times, should be emphasized here as an example of media studies analysis of the emerging phenomenon of self-tracking in amateur sport. Self-tracking is one of many processes mediated in everyday life, but due to the growing popularity of this type of services, it is becoming more and more popular not only among users, but also among theorists. S. Lombork and K. Frandsen view self-tracking as a communication phenomenon in three dimensions: the user and the tracking technology, the user and the self, and the user and a social network of peers. [21] They perceive the existence of several phenomena, e.g., the change from bodily to psychological experience through documentation, the importance of communicating with peers, motivating oneself and others. The results presented in this volume complement the existing explanations, penetrating deeper into structures and processes in order to answer the question of how in practice physical activity is mediated, not only through self-tracking, but also through other related processes.

The pace of changes taking place in amateur sport and in the world of new media, inspires taking a look into the future with the aim of forecasting social, political, and ethical challenges: "what we need may be more attempts at coherent descriptions and prescient diagnoses, and more willingness on the part of scholars in mediatization to offer some counsel on what could happen if we as a society collectively embrace this or that course of action in the future."[22]

The first trend that emerges from the research is the desaturation of physical activity shows that despite the growing diversity and availability of popular technologies, many individuals might give up technology to do sports as an end in itself, and to do it in a more conscious and controlled manner. Reflection on one's own well-being and the way it is shaped may result from the growing tendency to self-educate, taking care of oneself, one's own health, on which technologies do not necessarily have a good influence. It is relevant not only to the mechanisms of mediatization described in this volume, but also to the growing awareness of the negative impact of the electromagnetic field. Classification of a medical conditions, such as hypersensitivity to electromagnetic field (EMF), has been a breakthrough not only in the formal, legal, and medical aspects, but also in social, political, and economic sense. The increasing awareness of its negative implications may lead to limited use of unnecessary, additional technologies, while in the context of technologies necessary in everyday life, e.g., at work, the resignation from which would result in self-exclusion.

The second possible trend is the emergence of more diversified and advanced technologies, equipped with new sensors, actuators, and embedded technologies enabling to translate physical activity results into specific tasks during the workout. On the one hand, it concerns the development of specialized, dedicated, and highly sophisticated technologies, and on the other, the process of universalizing technologies, so that they integrate many functions and areas of life that are already subject to quantification. Also, an increasing popularity of not only wearable technologies, but also technologies closely adjacent to the body, e.g., electronic tattoos, which do not require carrying, charging and remembering about them, while processing a lot of data about the condition of our body, can be expected.

Moreover, datafication of sport, increasingly based on big data, which will contribute to an even greater growth of the importance of interactive and passive communication is predicted to occur. The further development of the Quantified Self movement may contribute to the possibility of achieving even higher levels of amateur activity efficiency but also its greater integration and alignment with other aspects of life. Thus, the informational value of each analyzed movement parameter will increase, raising the transformational potential of technology in sport.

It is also worth emphasizing that operating on huge amounts of sensitive, personal data generates numerous challenges: from technical, through cultural and social, political, psychological, to ethical and moral dimensions. Therefore, the question of one's own activity media saturation safety limits needs to be addressed. Based on the obtained results, it seems to be rather fluid and ambiguous. It is shaped differently for each individual case, enforcing the need for media literacy, and the continuous, multi-aspect updates, to maintain the awareness of the consequences of subjecting one's own life to mediatization.

METHODOLOGICAL CONCLUSIONS AND THE FUTURE OF RESEARCH ON MEDIA SATURATION OF EVERYDAY LIFE

The conducted research, integrating the quantitative and qualitative dimensions, allowed for capturing various dimensions of mediatization of physical activity. An introductory, pilot survey facilitated the study's initial arrangements and the direction for further qualitative research. That, in turn, allowed to broaden the perspective, penetrate deeper into usage issues and the processual dimension of media saturation, and to examine mechanisms of mediatization. The analysis demonstrates the media saturation parameter application in research practice, and outlines its importance in defining micromechanisms and mezzo-mechanisms of mediatization. It also justifies the growing importance of the technological dimension of contemporary media.

The advantages of measuring the spectrum and variations of the saturation degree undoubtedly include the possibility of illustrating the scale and size of the phenomenon, mapping individual mediated processes, comparing data, and tracking changes within particular measurement stages. The disadvantages of using the survey method of the quantitative aspects of media saturation, in addition to classical limitations of these methods in social sciences, undeniably lie in its exploratory and introductive character and limited measurement capabilities. However, it opens up the space for further conceptualizations and allows for measuring the quantitative aspects of saturation while using other tools to obtain statistical data, e.g., from tracking applications.

In terms of qualitative research, the chosen methods, mainly interviews and observations, allowed for obtaining data leading to the establishment of the basic mechanisms governing physical activity mediatization. Undoubtedly, there are many other methods that could deepen the analysis and reveal other existing mechanisms. Those could include diary study, participatory observations, and analysis of data from head-mounted video cameras, e.g., for the purposes of the stimulated recall method.

The conducted research was, to a much greater extent, focused on relationships between technologies, content, and human activity within their material and nonmaterial dimensions. It is worth noting that contemporary mediatization of physical activity occurs without the presence of traditional media.[23] It is actually "mediatization based on the 'coexistence' of individualization and global reach within a shared mediaspace."[24] Undoubtedly, this phenomenon is concerned with mediatization, and not just "extended mediation," typical for the mass media era;[25] with "reflexive" mediatization of private, everyday life of individuals using personal media by the way of "interlink their own interests and issues with those of the mass media."[26] Thus, the study chiefly focuses on deep mediatization, "elaborate mediatization of social life"[27] that permeates all levels on which an individual functions.

The third stage of the recommended analysis of mediatization should encompass the changes on the macro level, i.e., on the global level of cultures, societies, and markets, shaping up the living conditions of the contemporary humankind. Unquestionably, sport and physical activity are an important element of everyday life, characterized both by internal diversity and distinctiveness, as well as common practices resulting from, among others, the universality of the technologies used. Physical activity is the sphere of testing new solutions, intensifying their usage, as it is evidenced by, e.g., the popularity of the Quantified Self movement. On the other hand, it shows very strong individualism in terms of applied technologies and implemented mediated processes and is highly susceptible to reverse tendencies. The observed trends in modern amateur sport result not only from technological progress, financial and infrastructural accessibility of technology, and the level of social awareness (regarding the importance of movement, for example for health and appearance purposes), but also from fashion, both for sports as well as for technologies dedicated to active individuals, who embrace it as a lifestyle.[28] Young individuals are particularly susceptible to new trends and are willing to test new solutions, hence it is not surprising that the level of processual saturation in this age group is relatively high. The study should be replicated and adapted to other age groups: individuals older and even younger than those surveyed in this study.

The mechanisms governing the emergence of media saturation in previously unresearched groups remain an unverified area. These groups comprise of mainly professional athletes and it would be worth examining to what extent the media saturation of professional sport differs from the saturation of amateur sport. Another issue to explore could focus on media saturation in other regions (e.g., in less urbanized areas, in other cultural contexts etc.).

The view presented in this volume is synchronous, showing shifts in the present world (but not historical changes).[29] Meanwhile, it would be worth looking at the phenomenon in diachronic perspective by examining the changes that may occur when the researched young generation becomes mature enough to evaluate the changes in the mediatization mechanisms over a period of time. As previously stated, the emerging desaturation also enforces research of active sports individuals who have never used media technologies (non-users) and those who, due to the impact of technology, have completely given up physical activity and even demonstrate hostility toward it (anti-users).

There is also necessity to conceptualize other parameters of change as well, for example, those located outside of the media interior and the three-dimensional sphere of the user's technology-content-action relationship. The political, market, and cultural parameters of mediation of amateur sport still require exploration. Their examination would allow for capturing further mechanisms of change, located mainly at the mezzo and macro level.

An interesting issue to explore lies within the broadly understood mediatization of human relocation and movement stemming from ethnology, in which sport and exercises are only a part of a larger picture. Therefore, the spatial aspect of media saturation deriving from the location of the media in the environment of individuals doing sports (not only in gyms, fitness clubs, sport clubs), but in the broadly understood environment of active individuals should be investigated. The analysis of its changeability, degree, and mechanisms could be a significant contribution to the overall research on the mediatization of sport.

Since "media constitute as well as reproduce the world we live in,"[30] the variability of the media and their dual nature: productive and reproductive, result in the lack of a static and finite, closed and comprehensive theory that could correspond to different domains of life in general. The constant processing and transformation of relationships and changes in real life mean that any theory may turn out to be incomplete and, in some dimensions, become outdated in the near future. In particular, the methods of research on mediatization will need to be updated alongside the technological development and the saturation of subsequent activities with the mediated processes.

The evolution of mediatization, similar to other metaprocesses, is non-linear and thus it is characterized by interruptions, ruptures, and conflicting, dissonant moments.[31] Mediatization may also take a waveform course.[32] Media researchers must be constantly prepared for changes in the developed concepts, tested theories, and applied methods. They equally cannot omit signals indicating the beginnings of new processes, including important turns, in order to be able to capture their mechanisms in statu nascendi. Therefore, the subjects of the study should be individuals gradually isolating themselves from media technologies or individuals who have always abstained from them. In order to study not only what occurs, but also what does not take place, one should explore the subject of the forms of physical activities and sport disciplines that demonstrate the strongest resistance to media saturation and mediatization. One should also investigate technologies that are not used, in other words, technologies that are available but that do not find supporters. What mechanisms decide that they become rejected or abandoned technologies?

In addition to outlining new aspects and potential research populations to further media saturation analysis, the initiated research opens up opportunities for extending and modifying the concept itself, starting from the new measurement variants and the calculation of its quantitative dimension, to defining new features of the qualitative dimension research. Thus, the integration of the phenomenology—materialistic theory of mediatization, media ecology, and broadly understood medium theory combined with other interdisciplinary approaches would enrich the concept and enable its transposition to research on other spheres of everyday life. These could include broadly understood well-being, leisure, including travelling and recreation, nutrition, health, cultural activity, social and civic activity, family and home life. Work, education, entertainment, spiritual and religious life, and family life are the spheres that are currently subjected to intense mediatization. It results, among other elements, from a high degree of media saturation, especially processual saturation, as well as from the specificity of media saturation, that generates concrete mechanisms of change at all levels.

The specificity of media saturation forces the use of interdisciplinary research instruments. There is a need to constantly define them for the purpose of specific research and theories development. While contextualization of the research is a prerequisite to the exploration and explication of media saturation, it also requires defining the analyzed area, the field, or a certain sphere of life. Studies on media saturation can contribute to the development of media research so long as they use knowledge resources, and in some cases, methods from other science and humanities. This applies to social sciences as well as to other disciplines with which media studies intersect in the study of mediatization, inducing political sciences, psychology, sociology, physical culture, medicine, and theology, to name just a few. The integration of perspectives bears the possibility of revealing other mechanisms that develop in parallel and with the participation of media technologies.

Media saturation research is able to examine the processes conditioning the mediatization of contemporary life. It can explain the significance of adequate (i.e., sufficient and relatively optimal) quantitative and qualitative media saturation conditions for mediatization processes. Media technology users have access to a variety of options that can meet their everyday needs and expectations. Studies on the spectrum of media saturation explained the reason for physical activity media individualization and personalization, and the degree of the revealed saturation is a common technological factor that facilitates the occurrence of mediatization on the social level. On the other hand, technologies chosen by a larger group of users often generate a wider change due to the implementation of specific mediated processes en masse, which transform sport on the individual level during the initial stage of their use, and on the collective level as they popularize. Their intensity (implementation by a sufficient number of active individuals), and above all their specificity, condition mediatization.

Mediatization alone undergoes transformation, too. While new technology or content can generate change, participants are able to modify their activities in response to mediatization, which entails further consequences in the media sphere and various areas of life. Thus, mediatization enters a cycle in which desaturation is a natural step.

The media saturation study indirectly and partially explained the reasons behind the attempts to demediatize physical activity. It mainly occurs due to the loss of optimal quantitative indicators and selected qualitative properties pertaining to saturation, which is mainly process-based. Too many mediated processes, too far-reaching implications influencing physical activity, induce abstention from technology in sport, and sometimes determine negative assessment of technological saturation of life in other dimensions, too. In this context, the desaturation of physical activity can be seen as one of the processes initiating a broader change in the paradigm of media use in everyday life, characterized by retreat, isolation, criticism, and distancing, and thus initiating the incipient demediatization trend. Until now, demediatization has rarely been of interest to researchers. Reflection on demediatization takes place primarily within the institutional paradigm. It is noticed mainly in politics[33] and business,[34] and, to a very limited extent, within the context of everyday life.[35] The technological and cultural paradigms contribute to the understanding of the mechanisms governing the emergence of reverse tendencies, as well as peculiar mediatizing paradoxes. Demediatization, if seen from the perspective of traditional media, means only the renunciation of transformational power of the creation, distribution and consumption of media content. Meanwhile, demediatization on the material level encompasses demediatizion of life or its part in the artifactual and processual dimension, with the aim of making a change. Initially, the change takes place mainly at the individual level, although, similarly to mediated processes, its scale may give rise to concrete social consequences. Therefore, it is worth exploring both: the course and retransformation of various spheres of life caused by demediatization as well as the individual and social costs of such change.

The theory of mediatization is often seen as based on an assumption that individuals are continuously subjected to media influence, and thus to continuous and unceasing mediatization. Whether they use the media or not, as members of the society shaped by the media, individuals live in the mediatized culture. However, the scope, scale, mechanisms, and the implications of mediatization should be differentiated depending on its context. Depending on particular spatial and temporal circumstances, mediatization acquires different qualities. It is neither homogeneous, nor it is always equally intense, since it is not based on fixed, but dynamic mechanisms, some of which trigger reverse processual flows. Therefore, mediatization analysis should be nuanced, corresponding to the specific socio-media worlds and specific contexts with the inclusion of media saturation as well as desaturation; in other words, of saturated, oversaturated and undersaturated areas; media users' habits and non-users' habits.

"Not all the consumers will necessarily accept the experiences which are on offer, but the point about media saturation is that everyone, in modern societies, is obliged to respond in one way or another to what the mass media are doing."[36] Although over twenty years have passed since this statement was published, the era of new media has come, and media saturation has gained new meanings, the appeal for a response remains valid and also refers to the possibility of demediatizing the life of contemporary individuals.

> "That's why our future research aims at these phenomena of *de-mediatization* [emphasis in original] that in some cases turn out as de-optionalization, de-quantification and de-acceleration in others as forms of new regulatory interventions that also aim at installing some 'brakes" in the spread of unintended appropriation and its non-anticipative consequences."[37]

Emergent demediatization demands a multi-paradigmatic, transdisciplinary study,[38] and the area of everyday life, including physical activity, seen as its core topic since it constitutes a hot spot where tendencies and changes emerge, allowing for an examination of other aspects of everyday life.

Media saturation transforms, but also becomes a transformative entity of itself. By penetrating into objects of everyday use, the technology hybridizes the environment in an intensive manner. It facilitates a slow move toward a fully saturated, quantitively and qualitatively, everyday environment, in which the separation of what is online and offline becomes progressively blurred. The transparency of technology favors integration, however processes are likely to be noticed when it will not be possible to execute them. This raises the need for a deeper reflection on the accountability and the ethics of everyday life in the media environment integrated to that extent.

NOTES

1. Friedrich Krotz, "Media as a Societal Structure and a Situational Frame for Communicative Action: A Definition of Concepts," in *Critical Perspectives on the European Mediasphere,* eds. Ilija Tomanić Trivundža, Nico Carpentier, Hannu Nieminen, Pille Pruulmann-Venerfeldt, Richard Kilborn, Ebba Sundin and Tobias Olsson (Ljubljana: Faculty of Social Sciences: Založba FDV, 2011): 37.

2. Sonia Livingstone and Peter Lunt, "Mediatization: an Emerging Paradigm for Media and Communication Studies," in *Mediatization of Communication. Handbooks of Communication Science* (21), ed. Knut Lundby (Berlin: De Gruyter Mouton, 2014): 717.

3. Adam Greenfield, *Radical Technologies: The Design of Everyday Life* (London, New York: Verso Books, 2017), chapter available online: The Sociology of Smartphone, https://longreads.com/2017/06/13/a-sociology-of-the-smartphone/ (retrieved online).

4. Niels Ole Finnemann, "Mediatization Theory and Digital Media," *Communications* 36 (2011): 85.

5. Ernesto Ramirez, *The State of Self-Tracking*. http://quantifiedself.com/2013/03/the-state-of-self-tracking/ (retrieved online). Only 1 of the 300 surveyed respondents showed a high processual saturation degree, with a low technological saturation degree, which may indicate a measurement error.

6. James Miller, "The Fourth Screen: Mediatization and the Smartphone," *Mobile Media & Communication* 2.2 (2014): 212, 217.

7. Charles Leadbeater and Paul Miller, *The Pro-Am Revolution: How Enthusiasts are Changing our Society and Economy* (London: Demos, 2004).

8. Costas I. Karageorghis and Peter C. Terry, "The Psychological, Psychophysical, and Ergogenic Effects of Music in Sport: A Review and Synthesis," in *Sporting Sounds: Relationships between Sport and Music*, eds. Anthony Bateman and John Bale (London: Routledge, 2008).

9. Varoth Chotpitayasunondh and Karen M. Douglas, "How 'Phubbing' Becomes the Norm: The Antecedents and Consequences of Snubbing via Smartphone," *Computers in Human Behavior* 63 (2016).

10. Clifton Evers, "Masculinity, Sport and Mobile Phones," in *The Routledge Companion to Mobile Media*, eds. Gerard Goggin and Larissa Hjorth (London and New York: Routledge, 2014).

11. Paul Gilchrist and Belinda Wheaton, "New Media Technologies in Lifestyle Sport," in *Digital Media Sport: Technology, Power and Culture in the Network Society*, eds. Bret Hutchins and David Rowe (New York: Routledge 2013): 178.

12. Ibid.,181.

13. Kirsten Frandsen, "Mediatization of Sports," in *Mediatization of Communication*, ed. Knut Lundby (Berlin: Mouton de Gruyter, 2014). Kirsten Frandsen, "Sports Organizations in a New Wave of Mediatization," *Communication and Sport* (4) 2016.

14. Thomas Birkner and Daniel Nolleke, "Soccer Players and their Media Related Behaviour: A Contribution on the Mediatization of Sports, *Communication and Sport* 4 (2016).

15. Andrew C. Billings, *Olympic Media: Inside the Biggest Show on Television* (London, New York: Routledge, 2008).

16. David Rowe, "Media and Sport: The Cultural Dynamics of Global Games," *Sociology Compass* 3 (2009). David Rowe, "Global Media Sport: Flows, Forms and Futures," in *Sport, Media and Mega-events*, eds. Lawrence A. Wenner and Andrew C. Billings (London: Taylor & Francis, 2017).

17. Yair Galily and Ilan Tamir, "A Match Made in Heaven?! Sport, Television, and New Media in the Beginning of the Third Millennia." *Television & New Media* 15 (2014).

18. Gerard Goggin, "Sport and the Rise of Mobile Media," in *Digital Media Sport: Technology, Power and Culture in the Network Society*, eds. Brett Hutchins and David Rowe (New York: Taylor & Francis, 2013), 19–36.

19. Jimmy Sanderson, *It's a Whole New Ballgame: How Social Media is Changing Sports* (New York: Hampton Press, 2011).

20. Brett Hutchins, "Sport on the Move. The Unfolding Impact of Mobile Communications on the Media Sport Content Economy." *Journal of Sport & Social Issues* 38 (2014). Brett Hutchins, "Twitter Follow the Money and Look Beyond Sports." *Communication & Sport* (2) 2014. Brett Hutchins, and Janine Mikosza, "The Web 2.0 Olympics: Athlete Blogging, Social Networking and Policy Contradictions at the 2008 Beijing Games." *Convergence: The International Journal of Research into New Media Technologies* (16) 2010. Brett Hutchins and David Rowe, "Reconfiguring Media Sport for the Online World: An Inquiry into Sports News and Digital Media." *International Journal of Communication* (4) 2010.

21. Lombork, Frandsen, 1016.

22. Lynn Schofield Clark, "Mediatization: Concluding Thoughts and Challenges for the Future," in *Mediatized Worlds. Culture and Society in a Media Age*, eds. Andreas Hepp and Friedrich Krotz (Basingtoke: Palgrave Macmillan, 2014): 320.

23. As opposed to professional sport.

24. Niels Ole Finnemann, "The Internet and the Nordic Model of the Information Society," in *Sociedad de la Información y del Conocimiento en los Países Nórdicos: Semejanzas y Divergencias con el Caso Sspañol*, ed. Mariano Cebrian Herreros (Barcelona: Gedisa, 2009): 17. Postprint downloaded from: http://static-curis.ku.dk/portal/files/171652753/Finnemann_The_Internet_and_the_Nordic_model_of_the_Information_society.pdf.

25. Ibid., 17.

26. Frank Marcinkowski and Adrian Steiner, "Mediatization and Political Autonomy: A Systems Approach," in *Mediatization of Politics: Understanding the Transformation of Western Democracies.*, eds. Frank Esser and Jesper Strömbäck (London: Springer, 2014): 80.

27. Finnemann, ibid., 18.

28. Amanda DiFonzo, *Cyberbullying, Social Media & Fitness Selfies: An Evolutionary Perspective*, Master's Thesis, Brock University St. Catharines (Ontario: Brock University: St. Catharines, 2016): 3, http://dr.library.brocku.ca/bitstream/handle/10464/10433/Brock_DiFonzo_Amanda_2016.pdf?sequence=1 (retrieved online).

29. Norm Friesen and Theo Hug, "The Mediatic Turn: Exploring Concepts for Media Pedagogy, in *Mediatization: Concept, Changes, Consequences,"* ed. Knut Lundby (Frankfurt a. M.: Peter Lang, 2009): 70.

30. Mark Deuze, *Media Life* (Cambridge, MA: Polity, 2013), XI.

31. Andreas Hepp, *Cultures of Mediatization* (Cambridge, MA: Polity, 2013), 69.

32. Johan Fornäs, "Media Times. The Mediatization of Third-Time Tools: Culturalizing and Historicizing Temporality," *International Journal of Communication* 10 (2016): 20.

33. Speaking of "civic demediatization," J. Firmstone and S. Coleman focus on the content. However, they have mainly in mind the elimination of particular mass communication channels to favor digital channels; Julie Firmstone and Stephen Coleman, "Public Engagement in Local Government: the Voice and Influence of Citizens in Online Communicative Spaces," *Information, Communication & Society* 18.6 (2015): 687.

34. Esben Karmark, "Challenges in the Mediatization of a Corporate Brand: Identity-effects as LEGO Establishes a Media Products Company," *Media, Organizations and Identity,* ed. Mette Morsing (London: Palgrave Macmillan, 2010).

35. Johan Fornäs considers selected everyday reintegrating practices as a form of reintegration "challenging new media forms" described by Ovar Lofgren; Fornäs, ibid., 5223. Ovar Löfgren, "Domesticated Media: Hiding, Dying or Haunting," in *Strange Spaces: Explorations in Mediated Obscurity*, eds. Andre Jansson and Amanda Lagerkvist (London: Ashgate, 2009).

36. Andrew Tolson, *Mediations. Text and Discourse in Media Studies* (London: Arnold, 1996), 2.

37. Tilo Grenz, "Reflexive Mediatization. Insights into the Frictional Interplay between Customers and Providers," *KIT Working Paper* (2013), 17. http://pfadenhauer.org/blog/wp-content/uploads/2014/01/Working-Paper-Reflexivity-and-Frictional-Interplay.pdf (retrieved online).

38. An example here are Grenz's analyses that explain the mechanisms of online poker (acceleration, quantification, optimalization) and "emergent de-mediatization" laying at the foundations of the new model; Grenz, ibid., 7.

Appendix A

Usage of Media Technologies in Poland and Physical Activity of Poles

USAGE OF MEDIA TECHNOLOGIES IN POLAND

The research[1] showed that, in Poland, the highest number of Internet users (97%), wireless Internet users (88%), and social networks users (92%) is among young people aged 18–24. On average, they spend seventeen hours a week online, which is only 1 percent lower than in the 25–34 age group. It is worth noting that the highest percentage of Internet users from the 18–24 age group (50%) publish their own photos and films online since publishing is a paramount element of mediatization.

The percentage of Internet users per age group:

18–24:   97%
25–34:   95%
35–44:   80%
45–54:   60%
55–64:   39%
65+:   15%

The percentage of Internet users registered in social networks per age group:

18–24:   97%
25–34:   95%
35–44:   80%
45–54:   60%
55–64:   39%
65+:   15%

Average number of hours spent on the Internet weekly per age group:

18–24:   17 hours
25–34:   18 hours
35–44:   11 hours
45–54:   9 hours
55–64:   7 hours
65+:   7 hours

The percentage of Internet users who connect with the Internet with the use of mobile devices per age group:

18–24:   88%
25–34:   87%
35–44;   83%
45–54:   69%
55–64:   56%
65+:   62%

The percentage of Internet users who published photos or videos made by themselves during the past month per age group:

18–24:   50%
25–34:   40%
35–44:   15%
45–54:   13%
55–64:   18%
65+:   7%

The research[2] showed that population is technologically savvy. Moreover, their responses display a low resistance to technology. The highest number of all survey respondents (54%) among people in the 18–24 age group declare no fears related to using technologies. Only 3 percent of people aged 18–24 feel that technological changes are taking place too fast. It is the age group in which the most respondents (29%) state that they can't imagine life without access to the Internet and they represent the largest group of individuals who are passionate about new technologies (19%). Perhaps not surprisingly, they are aware of a significant impact of technology on their lives. None of the respondents said that they do not see such influence, which significantly differentiates that group from older respondents.

The percentage of respondents stating: "I'm not afraid of new technologies, new technologies are a chance for development" per age group:

18–24:   54%
25–34:   50%
35–44:   47%
45–54:   49%
55–64:   47%
65+:   48%

The percentage of respondents stating: "Technological changes are happening too quickly, you can't keep up with them" per age group:

18–24:   4%
25–34:   17%
35–44:   6%
45–54:   7%
55–64:   15%
65+:   24%

The percentage of respondents stating: "I can't imagne my life without access to the Internet" per age group:

18–24:   29%
25–34:   24%
35–44:   17%
45–54:   17%
55–64:   15%
65+:   7%

The percentage of respondents stating: "The development of technologies has not made a significant impact on my life" per age group:

18–24:   0%
25–34:   0%
35–44:   2%
45–54:   2%
55–64:   5%
65+:   10%

The percentage of respondents stating: "I'm passionate about new technologies, I'm interested in new developments and I want to have access to them as quickly as possible" per age group:

18–24:   19%
25–34:   17%
35–44:   13%
45–54:   6%
55–64:   5%
65+:   0%

Among other selection criteria, the place of residence of respondents was selected based on the highest number of Internet users in Poland who mainly populate cities with over 500,000 inhabitants.[3]

The percentage of Internet users in Poland according to the size of the place of residence:

Countryside:	56%
City up to 20,000 citizens:	60%
City 20,000–99,000 citizens:	61%
City 100,000–499,000 of citizens:	75%
City above 500,000 of citizens:	86%

Physical Activity of Poles

The research shows that engaging in sports is an activity done mainly by "young, well educated people, who are satisfied with their financial situation and live in cities."[4] Sixty-six percent of overall respondents did sports, with the number of respondents reaching 95 percent aged 18–24.

   While examining physical activity, research published hitherto did not link it only to traditional sports disciplines.[5] It encompassed, for example, physical activity registered during work, during time off work, in free time, and related to commuting—in Poland that was declared by 51.3 percent, 60 percent, and 71.8 percent of people above 15 years old for each area of activity respectively. Physical activity in free time and as part of commuting again turned out to be most popular among young people, reaching 37 percent among 15–19 years-old individuals and 28 percent amongst those aged 20–29 years old. Being active seem to be a domain of young people and the scope of various forms of physical activity including sports disciplines is high.

The percentage of respondents who declare doing sports during the last year (2013) per age group:[6]

18–24:	95%
25–34:	81%
35–44:	75%
45–54:	60%
55–64:	56%
65+:	35%

The percentage of respondents who engage in physical activity in their free time and as a means of commuting (2016) per age group:[7]

15–19:   37%
20–29:   28%
30–39:   17%
40–49:   13%
50–59:   15%
60–69:   12%

NOTES

1. Data presented below comes from the CBOS report. CBOS, "Internauci," *Komunikat z Badań CBOS* 90/2015 (retrieved online).

2. Data presented below comes from the Fundacja Orange report. Fundacja Orange, *Postrzeganie Internetu i Nowych Technologii w Polsce* (2015) (retrieved online).

3. CBOS, ibid.

4. CBOS, "Aktywność fizyczna Polaków," *Komunikat z Badań CBOS* 129/2013 (retrieved online).

5. Ministerstwo Sportu i Turystyki, "Poziom Aktywności Fizycznej Polaków," (Kantar Public, 2016) (retrieved online).

6. CBOS, ibid.

7. Ministerstwo Sportu i Turystyki, ibid.

Appendix B

Calculations of the Population Sample

Table Annex 2.1. Number of Wrocław residents with a distinction made for the sample age groups.

Wrocław Residents	Total	Women	Men
15–19	23678	11706	11972
20–24	30698	15306	15392
Total people aged 15–24	54376	27012	27364
Total of Wrocław residents	635759	339105	296654

Source: Local Data Bank of the Central Statistical Office of Poland

Wrocław's population statistics[1] show that in 2015 the city housed almost 636,000 residents, including 53.3 percent women (339,000) and 46.7 percent men (297,000). The number of people in the age group targeted in the survey reaches 54,400, including 23,700 individuals aged 15–19 and 30,700 aged 20–24. It means that people aged between 15 and 24 form 8.6 percent of the total number of Wrocław's residents. Within those age categories, the number of women and men is equal (the deviation from 50 percent of residents does not exceed 0.5 percent).

The number of residents of the Wrocław agglomeration reached 965,000.[2] When Wrocław's borders are extrapolated onto the entire Wrocław agglomeration, the estimated number of people from the age group of 15–24 reaches 82,000 (which corresponds with the size of the survey population sample).

Based on that assumption, only people who are physically active have been surveyed, which affected the population size significantly. The surveys collected from the nationwide population sample of Poles in 2012 show[3] that in the age group of 15–24, about 30 percent of the people regularly engage in physical activities. However, in recent years, doing sports has become increasingly trendy, and therefore an increase to 32 percent can be assumed.

Consequently, the population of physically active people in the Wrocław agglomeration aged 15–24 amounts to 26,300.

Since the population of women and men in the analyzed age groups is comparable, it should be noted that men have a higher ratio of engaging in regular physical activity (21,8 percent men vs. 18,9 percent women), it is necessary to include 4–5 percent (54.5 percent men and 45.5 percent women) more men in the survey sample. The gender division obtained in the designed survey sample reflects that ratio.

The population of individuals aged between 15 and 19 is smaller (43%) than those aged between 20 and 24 (57%), however the ratio of taking up regular physical activity is much higher among the former (39%) than the latter (24%). Based on that, it has been estimated that in the survey sample, about 55 percent should be people in the age group of 15–19. In the actual survey, people from the 19–24 cohort are over-represented. In a randomly selected sample of the above parameters, the level of trust would be 91 percent, with the error margin of 0.5. The sample was purposeful rather than random, therefore, in the strict statistical sense, it does not allow to draw conclusions about the entire population. However, due to population parameters, the presented results can be treated as highly probable, and sufficiently reliable as a starting point for qualitative research.

NOTES

1. Data presented below comes from the Local Data Bank of the Central Statistical Office of Poland.

2. Agencja Rozwoju Aglomeracji Wrocławskiej, "Aglomeracja-Wroclawska-w-liczbach," (retrieved online).

3. Data from the Local Data Bank of the Central Statistical Office of Poland.

Bibliography

Adolf, Marian T. "Clarifying Mediatization: Sorting through a Current Debate,"*Empedocles: European Journal for the Philosophy of Communication* 3.2 (2011): 153–75.

Adolf, Marian T. and Nico Stehr. "The Return of Social Physics?" in *The Technology of Information, Communication and Administration–An Entwined History*. Bern: Swiss Federal Archives, 2015. 1–9. https://www.researchgate.net/profile/Marian_Adolf/publication/274388297_The_Return_of_Social_Physics/links/551e85dc0cf29dcabb03fe0b.pdf (accessed June 30, 2018).

Agencja Rozwoju Aglomeracji Wrocławskiej. Aglomeracja-Wroclawska-w-liczbach." https://archive.is/AJRpV (accessed June 30, 2018).

Altheide, David and Snow Rober. *Media Logic*. Beverly Hills: Sage Publications, 1979.

Ammer, Christine and Dean S. Ammer. *Dictionary of Business and Economics*. New York, London: Macmillan, 1996.

Ang, Ien. *Living Room Wars. Rethinking Media Audiences*. London: Routledge, 1995.

Barker, Larry L. and Gordon Wiseman. "A Model of Intrapersonal Communication," *Journal of Communication* 16.3 (1966): 172–79.

Baudrillard, Jean. *Symbolic Exchange and Death*. London: Sage Publications, 1993.

Bennett, Andy. "Postmodernism," in Andy Bennett, *Culture and Everyday Life*. Thousand Oaks: Sage Reference, 2005. doi: http://dx.doi.org/10.4135/9781446219256.n2 (accessed March 14, 2018).

Berger, Peter L. and Thomas Luckmann. *The Social Construction of Reality: A Treatise in the Sociology of Knowledge*. London: Penguin, 1996.

Billings, Andrew C., *Olympic Media: Inside the Biggest Show on Television*. London, New York: Routledge, 2008.

Bolin Göran. *Media Generations: Experience, Identity and Mediatised Social Change*, London and New York: Routledge, 2016.

———. "The Rhythm of Ages: Analyzing Mediatization Through the Lens of Generations Across Cultures," *International Journal of Communication* 10 (2016): 5252–69.

Brown, Katrina Myrvang, Rachel Dilley and Keith Marshall. "Using a Head-mounted Video Camera to Understand Social Worlds and Experiences," *Sociological Research Online* 13(6), 1 (2008): 1–10.

Bull, Michael. "Investigating the Culture of Mobile Listening: From Walkman do iPod," in *Consuming Music Together: Social Collaborative Aspects of Music Consumption Technologies*, eds. Kenton O'Hara and Barry Brown. Heidelberg: Springer, 2006. 131–49.

———. "No Dead Air! The iPod and the Culture of Mobile Listening," *Leisure Studies* 24 (4) (2005): 343–55.

———."The World According to Sound Investigating the World of Walkman Users," *New Media & Society* 3 (2) (2001): 179–97.

CBOS. "Aktywność Fizyczna Polaków. Komunikat z Badań CBOS 129/2013," http://www.cbos.pl/SPISKOM.POL/2013/K_129_13.PDF (accessed June 30, 2018).

CBOS. "Internauci. Komunikat z Badań CBOS 90/2015." https://www.cbos.pl/SPIS KOM.POL/2015/K_090_15.PDF (accessed June 30, 2018).

Chotpitayasunondh, Varoth and Karen M. Douglas. "How 'Phubbing' Becomes the Norm: The Antecedents and Consequences of Snubbing via Smartphone," *Computers in Human Behavior* 63 (2016): 9–18.

Clark, Lynn Schofield. "Mediatization: Concluding Thoughts and Challenges for the Future," in *Mediatized Worlds. Culture and Society in a Media Age*, eds. Andreas Hepp and Friedrich Krotz. Basingtoke: Palgrave Macmillan, 2014. 307–23.

Contractor, Noshir, Peter Monge and Paul M. Leonardi. "Network Theory: Multidimensional Networks and the Dynamics of Sociomateriality: Bringing Technology Inside the Network," *International Journal of Communication* 5, 39 (2011): 682–720.

Couldry, Nick and Andreas Hepp. *The Mediated Construction of Reality*. Cambridge, MA: Polity, 2017.

Couldry, Nick. "Digital Storytelling, Media Research and Democracy: Conceptual Choices and Alternative Futures," in *Digital Storytelling, Mediatized Stories: Self-representations in New Media. Digital Formations*, ed. Knut Lundby. New York: Peter Lang Publishing, 2008. 41–60.

———. "Transvaluing Media Studies," in *Media and Cultural Theory*, eds. James Curran and David Morley. Abingdon: Routledge, 2005. 177–94.

———. "Mediatization or Mediation? Alternative Understandings of the Emergent Space of Digital Storytelling," *New Media & Society* 3 (2008): 373–91.

Creswell, John, W. *Research Design: Qualitative, Quantitative, and Mixed Methods Approaches*. Los Angeles: Sage Publications, 2009.

Deacon, David, and James Stanyer. "Mediatization: Key Concept or Conceptual Bandwagon?" *Media, Culture & Society* 36.7 (2014): 1032–44.

Deleuze, Gilles. *Negotiations 1972–1990*. New York: Columbia University Press, 1995.

Deloitte Digital. "Raport Strategiczny. Internet 2015/2016," http://iab.org.pl/wp-con tent/uploads/2016/06/Raport-strategiczny-Internet-2015_2016.pdf (accessed June 30, 2018).

Dempsey, Nicholas P. "Stimulated Recall Interview in Ethnography," *Qualitative Sociology* 33 (2010): 349–67.

Deuze, Mark, *Media Life*. Cambridge, MA: Polity, 2013.

Dewdney, Andrew and Peter Ride. *The Digital Media Handbook*. London: Routledge, 2013.

Dewey, Caitlin. "Are 'WiFi Allergies' a Real Thing? A Quick Guide to Electromagnetic Hypersensitivity," *The Washington Post,* August 31, 2015. https://www.washingtonpost.com/gdpr-consent/?destination=%2fnews%2fthe-intersect%2fwp%2f2015%2f08%2f31%2fare-wifi-allergies-a-real-thing-a-quick-guide-to-electromagnetic-hypersensitivity%2f%3f&utm_term=.b843bbfc562d (accessed June 30, 2018).

Dias, Marcos. "The Converging Worlds of 'Surfing the Web' and the Sport of Surfing" in A Scholarly Affair: Proceedings of the Cultural Studies Association of Australasia 2010 National Conference, eds. Baden Offord and Rob Garbutt. Lismore: Centre for Peace and Social Justice and the School of Arts and Social Science, 2011. 63–69.

DiFonzo, Amanda. "Cyberbullying, Social Media & Fitness Selfies: An Evolutionary Perspective." Master Thesis. Ontario: Brock University St. Catharines, 2016. http://dr.library.brocku.ca/bitstream/handle/10464/10433/Brock_DiFonzo_Amanda_2016.pdf?sequence=1 (accessed June 30, 2018).

Dobek-Ostrowska, Bogusława. *Komunikowanie Polityczne i Publiczne*. Warszawa: Wydawnictwo Naukowe PWN, 2007.

Drotner, Kirsten. "Boundaries and Bridges: Digital Storytelling in Education Studies and Media Studies," in *Digital Storytelling, Mediatized Stories*, ed. Knut Lundby. New York: Peter Lang, 2008. 61–81.

Eoin, Devereux. *Understanding the Media*. London: Sage Publications, 2007.

Evers, Clifton. "Masculinity, Sport and Mobile Phones," in *The Routledge Companion to Mobile Media*, eds. Gerard Goggin and Larissa Hjorth. London and New York: Routledge, 2014. 375–84.

———. "Researching Action Sport with a GoPro™ Camera: An Embodied and Emotional Mobile Video Tale of the Sea, Masculinity and Men-who-surf," in *Researching Embodied Sport: Exploring Movement Cultures. Routledge Research in Sport, Culture and Society*, ed. Ian Wellard. London: Routledge, 2015. 145–63.

Fetters, Michael D., Leslie A. Curry and John W. Creswell. "Achieving Integration in Mixed Methods Designs—Principles and Practices," *Health Services Research* 48.6pt2 (2013): 2134–56, https://www.ncbi.nlm.nih.gov/pmc/articles/PMC4097839/ (accessed June 30, 2018).

Finnemann, Niels Ole. "Mediatization Theory and Digital Media," *Communications* 36 (2011): 67–89.

———. "The Internet and the Nordic Model of the Information Society," in *Sociedad de la Información y del Conocimiento en los Países Nórdicos: Semejanzas y Divergencias con el Caso Español*, ed. Mariano Cebrian Herreros. Barcelona: Gedisa, 2009. 196–222. Postprint downloaded from: http://static curis.ku.dk/portal/files/171652753/Finnemann_The_Internet_and_the_Nordic_model_of_the_Information_society.pdf (accessed June 30, 2018): 1–22.

Firmstone, Julie, and Stephen Coleman. "Public Engagement in Local Government: the Voice and Influence of Citizens in Online Communicative Spaces," *Information, Communication & Society* 18.6 (2015): 680–95.

Floridi, Luciano. "A Look into the Future Impact of ICT on our Lives," *The Information Society* 23 (2007): 59–64.

Fornäs, Johan. "Media Times. The Mediatization of Third-Time Tools: Culturalizing and Historicizing Temporality," *International Journal of Communication* 10 (2016): 5213–32.

Frandsen, Kirsten. "Sports Broadcasting, Journalism and the Challenge of New Media." *MedieKultur: Journal of Media and Communication Research* 28 (53) (2012): 5–21.

———. *Tour De France: Mediatization of Sport and Place*, in *Sport, Media and Mega-events*, eds. Lawrence A. Wenner, Andrew C. Billings. New York: Routledge, 2017. 156–69.

———. "Sports Organizations in a New Wave of Mediatization." *Communication & Sport* 4 (4) (2016): 385–400.

———. "Mediatization of Sports," in *Mediatization of Communication*, ed. Knut Lundby. Berlin: Mouton de Gruyter, 2014. 525–34.

Friesen, Norm, and Theo Hug. "The Mediatic Turn: Exploring Concepts for Media Pedagogy," in *Mediatization: Concept, Changes, Consequences*, ed. Knut Lundby. Frankfurt a. M.: Peter Lang, 2009. 63–83.

Fundacja Orange. *Postrzeganie Internetu i Nowych Technologii w Polsce* (2015), http://www.orange.pl/ocp-http/PL/Binary2/2005128/4106503993.pdf (accessed June 30, 2018).

Galily, Yair, and Ilan Tamir. "A Match Made in Heaven?! Sport, Television, and New Media in the Beginning of the Third Millennia." *Television & New Media* 15 (2014). 699–702.

Gasperini, Kathleen. "Kodak Courage," *Mountain Sport and Living* (January–February 1999).

Gergen, Kenneth J. *The Saturated Self: Dilemmas of Identity in Contemporary Life*, New York: Basic Books, 1991.

Giddens, Anthony. *The Constitution of Society: Outline of the Theory of Structuration*, Berkeley: University of California Press, 1984.

Gilchrist, Paul and Belinda Wheaton. "New Media Technologies in Lifestyle Sport," in *Digital Media Sport: Technology, Power and Culture in the Network Society*, eds. Brett Hutchins and David Rowe. New York: Routledge, 2013. 169–87.

Glaser, Barney G. and Anselm L. Strauss. *Discovery of Grounded Theory: Strategies for Qualitative Research*. New Brunswick, NJ: Aldine Transaction, 1967.

Goggin, Gerard. "Sport and the Rise of Mobile Media," in *Digital Media Sport: Technology, Power and Culture in the Network Society*, eds. Brett Hutchins and David Rowe. New York: Taylor & Francis, 2013. 19–36.

Greenfield, Adam. "Radical Technologies: The Design of Everyday Life." London, New York: Verso Books, 2017, in *The Sociology of Smartphone*, https://longreads.com/2017/06/13/a-sociology-of-the-smartphone/ (accessed June 30, 2018).

Grenz, Tilo. "Reflexive Mediatization. Insights into the Frictional Interplay Between Customers and Providers," *KIT Working Paper*, 2013. http://pfadenhauer.org/blog/wp-content/uploads/2014/01/Working-Paper-Reflexivity-and-Frictional-Interplay.pdf (accessed June 30, 2018).

Gumpert, Gary, and Robert Cathcart. "A Theory of Mediation," in *Mediation, Information and Communication*, eds. Brent D. Ruben and Leah A. Lievrouw. New Brunswick: NJ: Transaction, 1990. 21–36.

———. "Media Grammars, Generations, and Media Gaps," *Critical Studies in Media Communication* 2.1 (1985): 23–35.

Hansen, Mark B. "Media Theory," *Theory, Culture & Society*, 23 (2006): 297–306.

Hepp, Andreas and Uwe Hasebrink. "Researching Transforming Communications in Times of Deep Mediatization: A Figurational Approach," in *Communicative Figurations, Transforming Communications—Studies in Cross-Media Research*, eds. Andreas Hepp, Andreas Breiter and Uwe Hasebrink. Cham: Palgrave McMillan, 2016. 15–48.

Hepp, Andreas, and Friedrich Krotz. "Mediatized Worlds: Understanding Everyday Mediatization," in *Mediatized Worlds: Culture and Society in a Media Age*, eds. Andreas Hepp and Friedrich Krotz. London: Palgrave, 2014. 307–23.

Hepp, Andreas. "Communicative Figurations. Researching Cultures of Mediatization," in *Media Practice and Everyday Agency in Europe*, eds. Leif Kramp, Nico Carpentier, Andreas Hepp, Ilija Tomanić Trivundža, Hannu Nieminen, Risto Kunelius, Tobias Olsson, Ebba Sundin and Richard Kilborn. Bremen: Edition Lumière, 2014. 83–99.

———. *Cultures of Mediatization*. Cambridge, MA: Polity, 2013.

———. "Differentiation: Mediatization and Cultural Change," *Mediatization: Concept, Changes, Consequences*, ed. Knut Lundby. New York: Peter Lang, 2009. 139–58.

———. "Researching 'Mediatised Worlds': Non-mediacentric Media and Communication Research as a Challenge." in *Media and Communication Studies Interventions and Intersections*, eds. Nico Carpentier, Ilija Tomanić Trivundža, Pille Pruulmann-Vengerfeldt, Ebba Sundin, Tobias Olsson, Richard Kilborn, Hannu Nieminen, Bart Cammaerts. Tartu: Tartu University Press, 2010. 37–48.

Hepp, Andreas, Andreas Breiter and Uwe Hasebrink. "Rethinking Transforming Communication: An Introduction," in *Communicative Figurations, Transforming Communications—Studies in Cross-Media Research*, eds. Andreas Hepp, Andreas Breiter and Uwe Hasebrink. Cham: Palgrave McMillan, 2016. 3–13.

Hepp, Andreas, Stig Hjarvard and Knut Lundby, "Mediatization: Theorizing the Interplay between Media, Culture and Society," *Media, Culture & Society* 37(2) (2015): 314–24.

Hjarvard, Stig. "The Mediatization of Society. A Theory of the Media as Agents of Social and Cultural Change," *Nordicom Review* 2 (2008):102–31.

———. *The Mediatization of Culture and Society*. London: Routledge, 2013.

Holmes, David. *Communication Theory: Media, Technology, Society*. Thousand Oaks: Sage Reference, 2005. doi: http://dx.doi.org/10.4135/9781446220733.n1 (accessed March 14, 2018).

Hunt, Robert W. G. "The Specification of Colour Appearance. I. Concepts and terms," *Color Research & Application* Vol. 2, 2 (1977): 55–68.

Hutchins, Brett. *Sport on the Move. The Unfolding Impact of Mobile Communications on the Media Sport Content Economy.* "Journal of Sport & Social Issues" 38 (2014): 509–27.

———. *Twitter Follow the Money and Look Beyond Sports.* "Communication & Sport" 2 (2014): 117–21.

Hutchins, Brett and Janine Mikosza, "The Web 2.0 Olympics: Athlete Blogging, Social Networking and Policy Contradictions at the 2008 Beijing Games." *Convergence: The International Journal of Research into New Media Technologies* (16) 2010: 279–97.

Hutchins, Brett, and David Rowe. "From Broadcast Rationing to Digital Plenitude; The Changing Dynamics of the Media Sport Content Economy," *Television and New Media* 4 (2009): 354–70.

———. "Reconfiguring Media Sport for the Online World: An Inquiry into Sports News and Digital Media." *International Journal of Communication* (4) 2010: 696–718.

———. *Sport Beyond Television: The Internet, Digital Media and the Rise of Networked Media Sport.* New York: Routledge, 2012.

Izcaray, Fausto. "Mass Media Saturation Conditions and Information Gaps in Venezuela." Doctoral Dissertation. Madison: University of Wisconsin, 1980.

Jansson, André and Magnus Andersson. "Mediatization at the Margins: Cosmopolitanism, Network Capital and Spatial Transformation in Rural Sweden," *Communications: the European Journal of Communication Research* 37(2) (2012): 173–94.

Jones, Janet and Lee Salter. *Digital Journalism.* Thousand Oaks: Sage Reference, 2012. doi: http://dx.doi.org/10.4135/9781446288634.n6 (accessed March 14, 2018).

Karageorghis, Costas I. and Peter C. Terry. "The Psychological, Psychophysical, and Ergogenic Effects of Music in Sport: A Review and Synthesis," in *Sporting Sounds: Relationships Between Sport and Music*, eds. Anthony Bateman and John Bale. London: Routledge, 2009. 13–36.

———. "Psychophysical Effects of Music in Sport and Exercise," in *Proceedings of the 2006 Joint Conference of the Australian Psychological Society and New Zealand Psychological Society.* Auckland: Australian Psychological Society, 2006, 415–19.

Karmark, Esben. "Challenges in the Mediatization of a Corporate Brand: Identity-Effects as LEGO Establishes a Media Products Company," *Media, Organizations and Identity,* ed. Mette Morsing. London: Palgrave Macmillan, 2010. 112–28.

Kember, Sarah and Joanna Zylinska. *Life after New Media: Mediation as a Vital Process.* Cambridge, MA: MIT Press, 2012.

Kopecka-Piech, Katarzyna. "Media Saturation as a Techno-social Phenomenon. Selected Examples of Smartphonisation in Social Life," in *Studia Kulturoznawcze* 3 (2017): 99-108.

Krotz, Friedrich and Andreas Hepp. "A Concretization of Mediatization: How Mediatization Works and why 'Mediatized Worlds' are a Helpful Concept for Empirical

Mediatization Research," in *Empedocles. European Journal for the Philosophy of Communication* 3 (2) (2013): 119–34.

Krotz, Friedrich. "Explaining the Mediatization Approach," *Javnost-The Public* 24.2 (2017): 103–18.

———. "From a Social Worlds Perspective to the Analysis of Mediatized Worlds," in *Media Practice and Everyday Agency in Europe*, eds. Leif Kramp, Leif Kramp, Nico Carpentier, Andreas Hepp, Ilija Tomanić Trivundža, Hannu Nieminen, Risto Kunelius, Tobias Olsson, Ebba Sundin and Richard Kilborn. Bremen: Edition Lumière, 2014. 69–82.

———. "Media as a Societal Structure and a Situational Frame for Communicative Action: A Definition of Concepts," in *Critical Perspectives on the European Mediasphere*, eds. Ilija Tomanić Trivundža, Nico Carpentier, Hannu Nieminen, Pille Pruulmann-Venerfeldt, Richard Kilborn, Ebba Sundin and Tobias Olsson. Ljubljana: Faculty of Social Sciences: Založba FDV, 2011. 27–39.

———. *Mediatisierung. Fallstudien zum Wandel von Kommunikation* 84. Wiesbaden: VS, 2007.

———. "Mediatization: A Concept with which to Grasp Media and Societal Change," in *Mediatization: Concept, Changes, Consequences*, ed. Knut Lundby. New York: Peter Lang Publishing, 2009. 21–40.

———. "Mediatization as a Mover in Modernity: Social and Cultural Change in the Context of Media Change," in *Mediatization of Communication. Handbooks of Communication Science* (21), ed. Lundby Knut. Berlin: De Gruyter Mouton, 2014. 131–61.

———. *Neue Theorien Entwickeln. Eine Einführung in die Grounded Theory, die Heuristische Sozialforschung und die Ethnographie Anhand von Beispielen aus der Kommunikationsforschung*. Köln: Halem, 2005.

———. "The Meta-process of Mediatization as a Conceptual Frame." *Global Media and Communication* 3 (3) (2007): 256–60.

Kubicek, Herbert. "Das Internet auf dem Weg zum Massenmedium? Ein Versuch, Lehren aus der Geschichte alter und Anderer neuer Medien zu Ziehen," in *Modell Internet? Entwicklungsperspektiven neuer Kommunikationsnetze*, eds. Raymund Werle and Christa Lang. Frankfurt a. M., New York: Campus Verlag, 1997.

Laurier, Eric. "Capturing Motion: Video Set-ups for Driving, Cycling and Walking," in *The Handbook of Mobilities*, eds. Peter Adey, David Bissell, Kevin Hannam, Pete Merriman and Mimi Sheller. Abingdon: Taylor & Francis, 2014. 493–502.

Laurier, Eric, Barry Brown and Moira McGregor. "Mediated Pedestrian Mobility: Walking and the Map App," *Mobilities* 11(1) (2016): 117–34.

Leadbeater, Charles and Paul Miller. *The Pro-Am Revolution: How Enthusiasts are Changing our Society and Economy*. London: Demos, 2004.

Leonardi, Paul M. "Digital Materiality? How Artifacts without Matter, Matter," *First Monday* 15.6 (2010).

Livingstone, Sonia and Peter Lunt. "Mediatization: an Emerging Paradigm for Media and Communication Studies," in *Mediatization of Communication. Handbooks of Communication Science* (21), ed. Knut Lundby. Berlin: De Gruyter Mouton, 2014. 703–24.

Lloyd, Mike. "On the Way to Cycle Rage: Disputed Mobile Formations," *Mobilities* 12(3) (2017): 384–404.

Löfgren, Ovar. "Domesticated Media: Hiding, Dying or Haunting," in *Strange Spaces: Explorations in Mediated Obscurity*, eds. Andre Jansson and Amanda Lagerkvist. London: Ashgate, 2009. 57–72.

Lomborg, Stine and Kirsten Frandsen. "Self-tracking as Communication," *Information, Communication & Society* 19.7 (2016): 1015–27.

Lundberg, Dan, Krister Malm and Owe Ronström. *Music, Media, Multiculture: Changing Musicscapes*. Svenskt Visarkiv, 2003. http://carkiv.musikverk.se/www/epublikationer/Lundberg_Malm_Ronstrom_Music_Media_Multiculture.pdf (accessed June 30, 2018).

Lundby, Knut. "Mediatization of Communication," in *Mediatization of Communication. Handbooks of Communication Science* (21), ed. Knut Lundby. Berlin: De Gruyter Mouton, 2014. 3–35.

———. "Notes on Interaction and Mediatization," in *Media Practice and Everyday Agency in Europe*, eds. Leif Kramp, Leif Kramp, Nico Carpentier, Andreas Hepp, Ilija Tomanić Trivundža, Hannu Nieminen, Risto Kunelius, Tobias Olsson, Ebba Sundin and Richard Kilborn. Bremen: Edition Lumière, 2014. 41–53.

Mackenzie, Susan Houge and John H. Kerr. "Head-mounted Cameras and Stimulated Recall in Qualitative Sport Research," *Qualitative Research in Sport, Exercise and Health* 4(1) (2012): 51–61.

Madianou, Mirca and Daniel Miller. *Polymedia*. 2010. http://blogs.nyu.edu/projects/materialworld/2010/09/polymedia.html (link does not exist: July 15, 2018).

Marcinkowski, Frank and Adrian Steiner. "Mediatization and Political Autonomy: A Systems Approach," in *Mediatization of Politics: Understanding the Transformation of Western Democracies*, eds. Frank Esser and Jesper Strömbäck. London: Springer, 2014. 74–89.

McLennan, Gregor. "Post-Marxism and the 'Four Sins' of Modernist Theorizing," *New Left Review* (218) 53 (1996): 53–74.

McLuhan, Marshall. "Understanding Media: The Extensions of Man." New York: Signet, 1964.

Meyrowitz, Joshua. "Understandings of Media," *ETC: A Review of General Semantics* 56.1 (1999): 44–52.

———. *No Sense of Place: The Impact of Electronic Media on Social Behavior*. New York: Oxford University Press, 1986.

Miller, James. "The Fourth Screen: Mediatization and the Smartphone," *Mobile Media & Communication* 2.2 (2014): 209–226.

Ministerstwo Sportu i Turystyki. "Poziom Aktywności Fizycznej Polaków" (Kantar Public, 2016). https://www.msit.gov.pl/download.php?s=1&id=11918 (accessed June 30, 2018).

Morley, David. "For a Materialist, Non–Media-centric Media Studies," *Television & New Media* 10.1 (2009): 114–116.

———. *Media, Modernity and Technology: The Geography of the New*. London: Routledge, 2007.

Morozov, Evgeny. "El Derecho a Desconectarse," *El Pais*. 2015. https://elpais.com/
elpais/2015/04/05/opinion/1428258905_239072.html (accessed June 30, 2018).

Morrell, Ernest. "Media Literacy," in *Encyclopedia of African American Education*, ed. Kofi Lomotey. Thousand Oaks: Sage Reference: 2010. doi: http://dx.doi
.org/10.4135/9781412971966.n158 (accessed March 14, 2018).

Morris, Merrill and Christine Ogan. "The Internet as Mass Medium," *Journal of
Computer-Mediated Communication*, Volume 1, Issue 4, 1 (1996): 39–50.

Mosby's Medical Dictionary. Liverport Lane: Elsevier, 2017.

Myrvang Brown, Katrina, Rachel Dilley and Keith Marshall. "Using a Head-mounted
Video Camera to Understand Social Worlds and Experiences," *Sociological Research Online* 13(6) (2008): 1–10.

Newell, Jay. "Revisiting Schramm's Radiotown: Media Displacemenet and Saturation," *Journal of Radio Studies* 1 (2007): 3–19.

Newell, Jay, Joseph J. Pilotta and John C. Thomas. "Mass Media Displacement and
Saturation," *The International Journal on Media Management* 4 (2008): 131–38.

Nowak, Kjell. "Medier Som Materiell och Mental Miljö," in Medierna i Samhället:
Igår, Idag, Imorgon, ed. Ulla Carlsson. Göteborg: Nordicom 1996. 159–76.

Nystrom, Christine. "Towards a Science of Media Ecology: The Formulation of Integrated Conceptual Paradigms for the Study of Human Communication Systems."
Doctoral Dissertation, New York: New York University, 1973.

O'Bannon, Loran. *Dictionary of Ceramic Science and Engineering*. New York, London: Springer, 2012.

O'Sullivan, Tim, Bryan Dutton and Philip Rayner. *Studying the Media. An Introduction*. London: Arnold, 1996.

Orlikowski, Wanda. "Using Technology and Constituting Structures: A Practice Lens
for Studying Technology in Organisations," *Organisation Science* 11 (4) (2000):
404–28.

Pallas, Josef. "Mediatization," in *The Sage Encyclopedia of Corporate Reputation*,
ed. Craig E. Carroll. Thousand Oaks: Sage Reference, 2016. doi: http://dx.doi
.org/10.4135/9781483376493.n175 (accessed March 14, 2018).

Pease, Roger W. Jr. *Merriam-Webster's Medical Dictionary*. Springfield, MA: Rebound by Sagebrush, 1995.

Peirce Sanders, Charles. *Collected Papers of Charles Sanders Peirce* Vol. 5, eds.
Charles Hortshorne and Paul Weiss. Cambridge: Harvard University Press,
1931–1958.

Postill, John and Brian Larkin. "Theorising Media and Change" (e-seminar, Melbourne, December 5–19, 2013), *Media Anthropology Network European Association of Social Anthropologists (EASA) E-Seminar Series*, http://www.media
-anthropology.net/file/postill_media_change.pdf (accessed June 30, 2018).

Postman, Neil. "The Reformed English Curriculum," in *High School 1980: The
Shape of the Future in American Secondary Education*, ed. Alvin Eurich. New
York: Pitman, 1970. 160–8.

Ramirez, Ernesto. *The State of Self-Tracking*. http://quantifiedself.com/2013/03/the
-state-of-self-tracking/ (accessed June 30, 2018).

Rooksby, John, Mattias Rost, Alistair Morrison and Matthew Chalmers. "Personal Tracking as Lives Informatics," in *Proceedings of the 32nd Annual ACM Conference on Human Factors in Computing Systems* (Toronto: ACM, 2014): 1165–66.

Rosa, Hartmut. *Social Acceleration: A New Theory of Modernity*. New York: Columbia University Press, 2013.

Rowe, David. "Global Media Sport: Flows, Forms and Futures," in *Sport, Media and Mega-events*. ed. Lawrence A. Wenner and Andrew C. Billings. London: Taylor & Francis, 2017. 699–701.

———. "Media and Sport: The Cultural Dynamics of Global Games," *Sociology Compass* 3 (2009). 543–58.

———. *Sport, Culture, and The Media: The Unruly Trinity*. Maidenhead: McGraw-Hill Education 2003.

Rusin-Dybalska, Renata. "Nowy Wymiar Komunikowania Politycznego na Przykładzie Języka Prezydenta Czech Miloša Zemana," *Rozprawy Komisji Językowej ŁTN Z*. 62 (2016): 117–30.

Sanderson, Jimmy. *It's a Whole New Ballgame: How Social Media is Changing Sports*. New York: Hampton Press, 2011.

Schmidt, Siegfried J. "Media Philosophy—A Reasonable Programme?" in *Philosophy of the Information Society*. 30th Wittgenstein Symposium. Frankfurt u. M.: Ontos, 2007. 89–105. http://wittgensteinrepository.org/agora-ontos/article/down load/2096/2305 (accessed June 30, 2018).

Schutz, Alfred, and Thomas Luckmann. *The Structures of the Life World*. Evanston, IL: Northwestern University Press, 1973.

Sherry, John, L. "Media Saturation and Entertainment-education," *Communication Theory* 2 (2002): 206–24.

Silverstone, Roger and Leslie Haddon, "Design and the Domestication of Information and Communication Technologies: Technical Change and Everyday Life," in *Communication by Design: The Politics of Information and Communication Technologies*, eds. Robin Mansell and Roger Silverstone. Oxford, UK: Oxford University Press, 1996. 206–24.

Silverstone, Roger. *Why Study the Media?* London: Sage Reference, 1999. doi: http://dx.doi.org/10.4135/9781446219461 (accessed March 14, 2018).

———. "The Sociology of Mediation and Communication," in *The Sage Handbook of Sociology*, eds. Craig Calhoun, Chris Rojek and Bryan Turner. London: Sage Reference, 2015. doi: http://dx.doi.org/10.4135/9781848608115.n11 (accessed March 14, 2018).

———. "Complicity and Collusion in the Mediation of Everyday Life," *New Literary History* 4 (2002): 761–80.

Simondon, Gilbert. *Du Mode des Objects Techniques*. Paris: Aubier, 1989.

Sorokin, Pitirim A. *Society, Culture, and Personality, Their Structure and Dynamics*. New York, London: Harper & Brothers Publishers, 1947.

Spinney, Justin. "A Chance to Catch a Breath: Using Mobile Video Ethnography in Cycling Research," *Mobilities* 6(2) (2011): 161–82.

Strate, Lance. *Echoes and Reflections. On Media Ecology as a Field of Study*. Cresskill, NJ: Hampton Press, 2006.

Strauss, Anselm. "A Social World Perspective," *Studies in Symbolic Interaction* 1.1 (1978): 119–28.

Sullivan, John L. "Mass Consumption," in *The Sage Glossary of the Social and Behavioral Sciences*, ed. John L. Sullivan. Thousand Oaks: Sage Reference, 2009. doi: http://dx.doi.org/10.4135/9781412972024.n1540 (accessed March 14, 2018).

Thompson, Glen. *From the Water to the Web: Surfing, Self, and the New Media in South Africa*. 2013. http://writingsurfinghistory.org.za/histories (accessed June 30, 2018).

Thorpe, Holly. *Transnational Mobilities in Action Sport Cultures*. Basingstoke: Palgrave Macmillan, 2014.

Thrift, Nigel. "Movement-space: The Changing Domain of Thinking Resulting from the Development of New Kinds of Spatial Awareness," *Economy and Society* 33(4) (2004): 582–604.

Todd, Gitlin. "Supersaturation, or, The Media Torrent and Disposable Feeling," in *Living in the Information Age*, ed. Erik P. Bucy. Belmond: Wadsworth Thomson, 2005. 13–70.

Tolson, Andrew. *Mediations. Text and Discourse in Media Studies*. London: Arnold, 1996.

Toffler, Alvin. *The Third Wave*. New York: Bantam Books, 1980.

Urbański, Mariusz. "O Rozumowaniach Abdukcyjnych," in *Propositiones*, eds. Tomasz Mróz and Mariusz Sieńko. Zielona Góra: Instytut Filozofii Uniwersytetu Zielonogórskiego, 2005. 143–50.

Van Dijck, José. "Datafication, Dataism and Dataveillance: Big Data between Scientific Paradigm and Ideology," *Surveillance & Society* 12(2) (2014): 197–208.

Vauquelin, Louis Nicolas and G. L. Brismontier, *Dictionary of Chemistry: Containing the Principles and Modern Theories of the Science, with its Application to the Arts, Manufactures, and Medicine*. New York: G&C&H Carvill, 1830.

WHO, *Physical Activity* (n.d.) http://www.who.int/ncds/prevention/physical-activity/en/ (accessed June 30, 2018).

Williams, Raymond. *Television: Technology and Cultural Form*. London: Routledge, 1990.

Index

213

About the Author

Katarzyna Kopecka-Piech is doctor of Humanities, new media researcher, and assistant professor at the University of Wroclaw, Institute of Journalism and Social Communication. She specializes in research on new technologies, mediatization of everyday life, media convergence, and media innovation. Previously, she was a postdoctoral scholar at the University of Oslo, Norway and at the Södertörn University, Sweden. She collaborated as a researcher with, among others, the University of Oxford, United Kingdom and the University of Physical Education in Wroclaw, Poland. She is a leader of the academic projects at Academia Europaea Wrocław Knowledge Hub, where she organizes international seminars on mediatization research. She is also involved as adviser and expert for public institutions and research agencies in Poland and the Czech Republic.